# First Aid

*Titles of related interest:*

G J Ebrahim: *Breast Feeding: the Biological Option*
G J Ebrahim: *Child Care in The Tropics*
G J Ebrahim: *Child Health in a Changing Environment*
G J Ebrahim: *Paediatric Practice in Developing Countries*
G J Ebrahim: *Practical Mother and Child Health in Developing Countries*
G J Ebrahim: *Care of the Newborn in Developing Countries*
G J Ebrahim: *Handbook of Tropical Paediatrics*
David Morley and Margaret Woodland: *See How They Grow*
Jean Ritchie: *Nutrition and Families*
Muriel Skeet: *Family Care*
Caroline Uddoh: *Nutrition*
David Werner: *Where There Is No Doctor*

# First Aid

For Community Health Workers
in Developing Countries

**MURIEL SKEET**

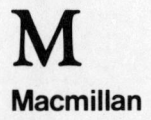

**M**
Macmillan

© Muriel Skeet 1984

All rights reserved. No part of this publication
may be reproduced or transmitted, in any form
or by any means, without permission

First published 1984 by
THE MACMILLAN PRESS LTD
London and Basingstoke
Companies and representatives
throughout the world

Printed in Hong Kong

ISBN 0-333-34710-2
ISBN 0-333-36385-X    Pbk

# Contents

Preface ... vii
Acknowledgements ... viii
Introduction ... ix

1. What to Find Out and What to Look For when Someone has an Accident or Becomes Ill Suddenly ... 1
2. What to Do when Someone Cannot Breathe Properly: Respiratory (breathing) and cardiac (heart) emergencies ... 9
3. What to Do when Someone has a Bad Cut or Wound ... 17
4. What to Do when Someone is Burned or Scalded ... 26
5. What to Do when Someone Cannot be Woken Up ... 29
6. What to Do when Someone Swallows Poison or is Poisoned by a Sting or Bite ... 32
7. What to Do when Someone has a Belly Pain (Stomach Ache) ... 40
8. What to Do when a Pregnant Woman Becomes Ill: Avoiding illness during pregnancy ... 47
9. What to Do when a Pregnant Woman Goes into Labour ... 53
10. What to Do when Someone has a Fit ... 62
11. What to Do when Someone is Affected by Great Heat or Cold ... 67
12. What to Do when Someone Breaks a Bone ... 70
13. What to Do when Something is Wrong with the Eye, the Ear, the Nose, or the Mouth ... 81
14. How to Take a Patient to Medical Help ... 85

Appendix I: How to Prevent Accidents and Poisonings ... 94
Appendix II: How to Use some of the Medicines Mentioned in this Book ... 98
Appendix III: How to Teach what is in this Book: Addresses from which Teaching Materials can be Obtained ... 99

Index ... 103

# Preface

Community health care addresses the main health problems in the community, providing promotive, preventive, curative and rehabilitative services accordingly. By its very nature, therefore, community health care includes the prevention of accidents as well as the prevention of disease; it includes the speedy healing of wounded flesh and broken bones as well as the cure of illness; and it includes the prevention of death and disability from accidents as well as the prevention of those consequences from malnutrition and infections.

In recent years much discussion has taken place of many important issues involved in attaining 'Health for All by the Year 2000'. From these have risen questions concerning vital debatable points such as the kind of basic training members of the health team should receive and how to incorporate individuals and families into that team so that they can become full partners in their own health and welfare development. The knowledge and skills inherent in preventing accidents and carrying out emergency procedures have been recognised as essential components of the former and important contributions to the latter.

All countries of the world have members of their population of all ages who are crippled or deformed for life as a result of accidents on the road, in the home or at work or school. Many old people in our midst are disabled and therefore dependent, because of unfortunate incidents in their earlier lives which could have been either prevented or dealt with more competently when they occurred. And everyone who has worked in a hospital in a developing country will know the horror of admitting to paediatric wards, hundreds of small children who have suffered severe, painful burns because families have not adequately protected the evening fires or boiling cooking pots. Gross and life-long disfigurement and disability or even death are not unusual consequences. Every year in every country of the world, therefore, lives are blighted or lost unnecessarily, just because no one near to hand has known what to do in an emergency.

Many threatened lives can be saved and the quality of saved lives restored—or even improved—if the right treatment is given at the right time, at the right place, by the right persons. This means the carrying out of correct emergency procedures by trained and accessible members of the community at the site of the accident—immediately.

This book is one attempt to help this to happen.

*Muriel Skeet*
*London, July 1983*

# Acknowledgements

I am most grateful to the many people who have made the production of this book possible.

First, to the British Red Cross Society and the League of Red Cross Societies, who, during my years with them, afforded me opportunities to see for myself the outstanding and universal need for the knowledge and skills of First Aid. I am also indebted to them for permission to interpret or paraphrase some of their published and unpublished material.

I acknowledge with very many thanks, permission to adapt some of the text produced by the Division of Health Manpower Development, World Health Organization, Geneva, in *The Primary Health Care Worker* (Revised Edition), and by David Werner in *Where There is No Doctor*.

For material I have used in Chapters 1, 2, 3, 4, 12 and 14, I would like to thank Blackwell Scientific Publications (London and Oxford) for their generous permission to reproduce this from *Emergency Procedures and First Aid for Nurses*, which I edited for them in 1981.

Finally, I thank all nurses, doctors, health educators and others who, over the years, and in many countries of the world, have shared with me their knowledge and experiences in providing first aid and carrying out emergency procedures skilfully and efficiently. To each one I extend my warm thanks and appreciation.

*Muriel Skeet*
*London, 1983*

# Introduction

This book on first aid is written primarily for community health workers in developing countries.

It is assumed that each will have already received some training in primary health care, will understand the most commonly used terms and be able to perform certain curative procedures, such as those included in the revised publication of the World Health Organization, *The Primary Health Worker*.[1] It is also assumed that each health worker has access to some form of pharmacopoeia (even if it is only a few sheets of paper), which he can consult for guidance on the dosage and administration of essential drugs.

In some instances the publication itself may be used as a source of reference. Under other circumstances it may be a teaching aid, and the text has been deliberately written in the second person to facilitate its use as an instruction manual. However, because culture, customs, habits, practical taboos and even specific accidents vary from one country to another, it is not possible to write a book which can be used by the whole world without adaptation. It is suggested, therefore, that this publication should be adapted according to local situations, flora, fauna and history. Some examples, such as the use of plants in traditional medicines, are given in the following pages, but there will be many other changes and amendments necessary which only local people will know and can make. Measurements given in the text will also need to be changed to local ones. This is particularly important in relation to medicines and lotions, and also to the making up of fluids such as normal saline or rehydration fluid.

As far as teaching is concerned, again traditional methods should be used: among rural people this is likely to include oral practices. If appropriate, use should be made of story-telling, parables, plays, songs, riddles and local proverbs. Differences in customs, even between next-door villages, are reflected in both the form and content of traditional stories. These should be followed and stories composed to include widely held knowledge, moving on to the action which one hopes to teach. If it conflicts with current beliefs new teaching will simply be ignored or laughed at.

When producing pictures for learning purposes, it may be borne in mind that tests have shown that photographs from which the background has been removed are the easiest for people to assimilate: these are frequently used in successful advertising all over the world. The simple line drawings in this book may also be easily reproduced either on a chalk board or flip chart.

The most important development of any country is the development of its people. People can be a nation's greatest asset and self-help is a key factor in human development. But in order to be self-reliant, knowledge has to be acquired, skills have to be learned and some attitudes have to undergo change. The rural health worker today finds himself with a major responsibility to inform, explain, guide, advise and generally assist his community and all families and individuals in it, to mutual development.

This publication is offered as a small contribution to help him in that important and life-saving responsibility.

M.S.

---

[1] *The Primary Health Worker: Working Guide: Guidelines for Training: Guidelines for Adaptation.* WHO, Geneva, 1980 (revised edition).

# 1. What to Find Out and What to Look For when Someone has an Accident or Becomes Ill Suddenly

## What first aid is

First aid is the treatment given when an accident or sudden illness occurs. The treatment is carried out by using whatever materials or equipment happen to be available at the time.

First aid is the treatment given until the patient can be removed to a first aid post, health centre, clinic or hospital or until more skilled help is available.

First aid is the emergency care given:

(1) to keep the injured or ill person alive;
(2) to prevent his condition from becoming worse;
(3) to help him to recover.

## Emergency care

The order for giving emergency care is:

(1) look at the general situation quickly;
(2) decide what is wrong and how severe or dangerous the injury is;
(3) give the appropriate first aid;
(4) notify your supervisor and arrange transport to hospital or health centre;
(5) give follow-up care during the journey.

## 1. Looking at the situation

The amount of time spent on this will depend upon answers to:

- how obvious is the injury or illness?
- how threatening to life is the injury or illness?
- how much do you already know about the person who is injured or ill?
- how threatening to life is the surrounding area (e.g. a room filled with poisonous fumes; nearby crocodiles, etc.)?

*Observation*

When you arrive at the scene of an accident or sudden illness, you must quickly sum up the general circumstances. If the cause is obvious, this may take only a few minutes. It is a particularly important thing to do if the casualty is unconscious and alone. Remember that an emergency may involve more than one person (e.g. an outbreak of food-poisoning or a motor-car crash).

Looking quickly and keenly can help you to decide what is likely to be wrong and what you are going to have to do. For example, if you find someone lying at the foot of a tree from which the fruits are being picked, you will know that the person is likely to have injured his muscles, bones or head. He may also be bleeding inside his body (internally). Drowning, electric shock, poisonous gases, will mean a breathing (respiratory) emergency. Fire and smoke will mean that you are likely to need your knowledge of how to treat burns and also how to assist a person to breathe.

*History of the accident or illness*

Not all causes of injuries and illnesses, however, can be seen and you may have to question the injured or ill person, his companions or the people standing by. If the patient is conscious, the history of the incident (the story of what happened), can be collected by direct questioning. For example, ask him 'What happened?' If he is unconscious or in no state to answer questions, the history may be taken from someone else who actually saw what happened. In this case it will be necessary to limit the story and to make it very clear that you want only relevant facts, and that you want them quickly. People often *want* to talk when they have seen an accident happen, because that relieves their own feelings of shock and worry.

## First Aid

### History of the patient

In order to find out what to do, it is necessary to obtain information about the patient's condition. This is called the patient's history. You should always ask direct questions such as 'What do you feel?' and not ask questions which suggest an answer, such as 'Do you feel faint?' Obviously, questioning and finding out what happened must not be allowed to delay you in getting on with the first aid which is necessary (such as getting someone who has stopped breathing to breathe again, and trying to stop any bleeding which you see). But a quick gathering of facts and a speedy assessment of what has happened will help you to decide what you must do first and also what you must *not* do.

### 2. Determining what is wrong and how severe or dangerous it is

#### Nature and severity of the emergency

The *nature* of the emergency means the type of emergency, such as cardiac—an emergency of the heart. Injury can be external damage—such as a cut leg which you can see, or it may be internal damage—such as a crushed stomach (belly), or liver—which you cannot see. Sometimes there are both. For example, severe injuries which you can see, may lead to a breathing and heart emergency which you cannot see. You must be able to recognise the signs and symptoms of these conditions you cannot see, because they also will require urgent treatment.

The *severity* of an emergency means how much it threatens life. For instance, while an ankle may be severely sprained, it will not kill and therefore is not a major injury. Your decisions concerning what should receive attention first, and what treatment should be given, will be based upon this kind of knowledge.

#### Examination of the patient

To find out the nature and the severity of an illness or injury, you should examine the patient in an orderly manner. First check:

- breathing (listen and look at the rise and fall of his chest if necessary);
- colour of skin (for dark-skinned people, note the palms of the hands, the soles of the feet and the lips);
- circulation of blood (by taking the pulse);
- pupils of the eyes (whether large or small and whether they change in light).

These signs give you vitally important information. For example, if breathing has stopped it means that the lungs have stopped working, and that you must get them going again quickly (see page 9). If you cannot feel a pulse, it may mean that the heart has stopped pumping blood and you must get that working again (see page 14). When both heart and lungs have stopped this is called cardio-pulmonary arrest (see page 14). Both these conditions mean death for the patient if they are not treated *at once*.

#### Check for severe bleeding

Bleeding is obvious when it occurs from outside (external) wounds or parts on the body you can see. It may not be obvious if it occurs under clothing or from a party of the body which is facing the ground. You must consider the possibility of serious bleeding which you cannot see (internal). Then there may be only signs and symptoms of severe shock (see pages 6–7).

An excessive loss of blood can cause severe shock which can kill within only a few minutes. Severe bleeding must therefore be dealt with immediately (see pages 17–18).

#### Check for poisoning

Some poisons can also cause death almost immediately. Poisoning can occur by swallowing certain chemicals, or by taking a very large amount of medicines, pills, capsules or other drugs. According to the amount and type taken, quick treatment may mean the difference between life and death. An indication of poisoning may be given by empty medicine or poison bottles or containers, or there may be burns and stains in and around the mouth.

Local insects, reptiles, etc., which are poisonous will probably be known, and fang marks made by poisonous snakes will be obvious. Local witches' brews should also be thought of as a source of poisoning.

#### Check for shock

Shock is caused by not enough blood getting pumped round the body. If the brain does not get enough, death can occur very quickly. This condition, therefore, requires very quick action (see pages 6–7).

## Check parts of the body

Look carefully and quickly at each part of the body, in the following order:

- head;
- neck;
- chest;
- abdomen (stomach or belly);
- back;
- arms, hands, fingers;
- legs, feet, toes.

Look for:

- signs of internal damage to organs (swelling and darkening of the skin);
- burns;
- wounds;
- fractures (broken bones);
- dislocations (bone put out of place);
- sprains;
- strains;
- bruising.

## Check when the emergency is a sudden illness and another condition is not due to injury

Emergency conditions can arise from many causes. When the exact cause is not obvious (e.g. a miscarriage in a pregnant woman), think of each body system in turn, making careful note and use of what the patient says, as well as his normal or abnormal functioning (e.g. notice whether speaking is difficult or his speech is slurred).

Body systems include:

- the cardio-pulmonary system (heart and lungs);
- the vascular system (circulation of blood and its vessels—arteries and veins and capillaries);
- the urinary system (kidneys, bladder and the passing of water);
- the digestive and excretory system (stomach, liver, gall-bladder, bowel (or gut) and the passing of stools (faeces));
- the reproductive system (including the genitals and organs used in intercourse and nourishing an unborn baby);
- the musculo-skeletal system (muscles and bones);
- the skin.

## Important signs and symptoms

A symptom is a change or difference in normal functioning of a person that indicates disease, injury or illness. The patient experiences a symptom. Examples are dizziness, nausea, pain and numbness.

A sign is a change or difference in the normal functioning of a person that other people can see and measure. Examples are a change in the colour of the skin, in the temperature, pulse or breathing (Fig. 1.1).

---

**TEMPERATURE**

There are two kinds of thermometer scales. Centigrade (C.) and Fahrenheit (F.).
Either can be used to measure a person's temperature.

Here is how they compare:

**CENTIGRADE**
This thermometer reads 40°C.
(Forty degrees Centigrade)

34 35 36 37 38 39 40 41 42

Too low | NORMAL | Some fever | High fever

92 94 96 98 100 102 104 106 108

**FAHRENHEIT**
This thermometer reads 104° F.
(104 degrees Fahrenheit)

---

**PULSE OR HEARTBEAT**

For a person at rest:
- ADULTS .......... 60–80 beats per minute is normal.
- CHILDREN ........ 80–100
- BABIES .......... 100–140

For each degree Centigrade (°C.) of fever, the heartbeat usually increases about 20 beats per minute.

---

**RESPIRATION**

For a person at rest:
- ADULTS AND LARGE CHILDREN ... 12–20 breaths per minute is normal.
- CHILDREN ........ up to 30 breaths per minute is normal.
- BABIES .......... up to 40 breaths per minute is normal.

---

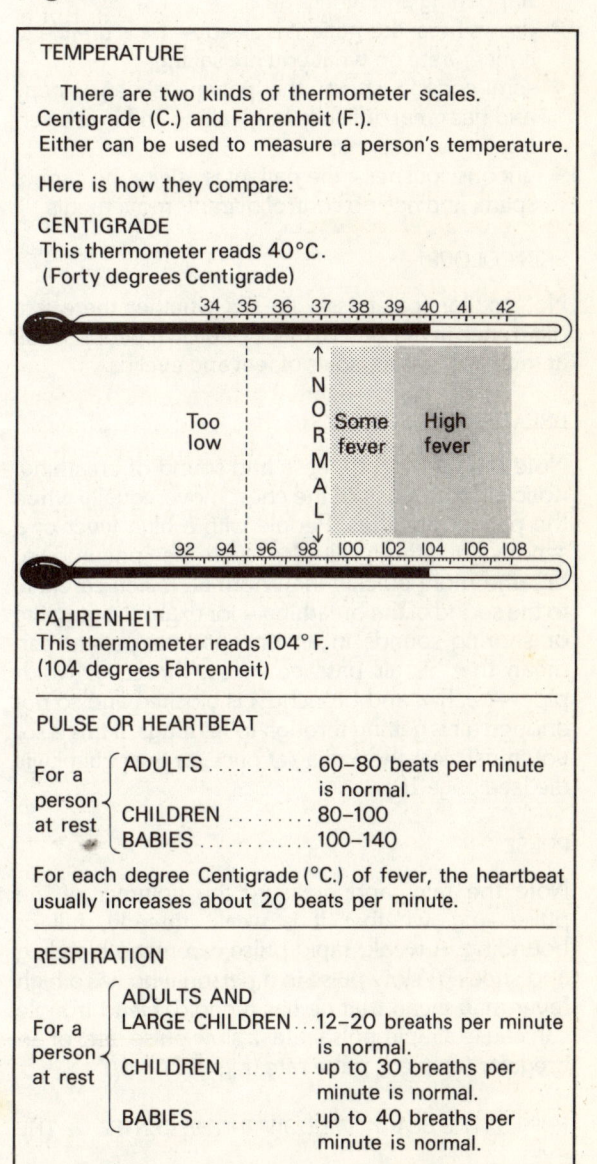

*Fig. 1.1 Collecting information on vital signs*

The following description of signs and symptoms should help you to determine the type and severity of the emergency with which you are dealing.

STATE OF CONSCIOUSNESS (BEING AWAKE AND AWARE)

Levels of consciousness may include:

- alertness: the patient can speak, answers questions and feels pain;
- lethargy: the patient is awake, but answers questions slowly—he may be confused about what is happening and where he is;
- drowsiness: the patient is sleepy—he is unable to concentrate on what you are saying;
- semi-consciousness: the patient is very sleepy and has great difficulty in speaking and in answering your questions;
- unconsciousness: the patient is asleep, he cannot speak and has no control over his movements.

SKIN COLOUR

Note pallor (paleness). To see whether there is a difference in the skin of black or brown people, look at their lips, palms, soles of feet and eyelids.

BREATHING (RESPIRATION)

Note the rate, depth, ease and sound of breathing; notice if both sides of the chest move equally when the patient breathes. People with a high fever or a serious breathing illness, such as pneumonia, breathe more quickly than normal. Listen carefully to the sound of the breathing—for example, gurgling or snoring sounds in an unconscious patient can mean that his air passage (nose, throat, or windpipe—trachea and bronchus) is blocked and so not enough air is getting through to his lungs. If this is so, you must clear the airway at once, or the patient will die (see page 10).

PULSE

Note the rate, and measure the volume, of the pulse—e.g. whether it is weak, thready, full or bounding. A weak, rapid pulse can mean bleeding and shock. A slow pulse in a person who has a high fever may mean that he has typhoid. Heart trouble can cause a rapid pulse rate, a slow pulse rate, or an irregular (uneven) pulse rate (Fig. 1.2).

PUPILS (THE BLACK 'WINDOW' IN THE CENTRE OF THE EYE)

When exposed to light, pupils usually constrict (get

---

Counting the pulse

1. Have a watch with a second-hand in front of you.
2. Place two fingers of your right hand above the patient's wrist as indicated on the drawing.

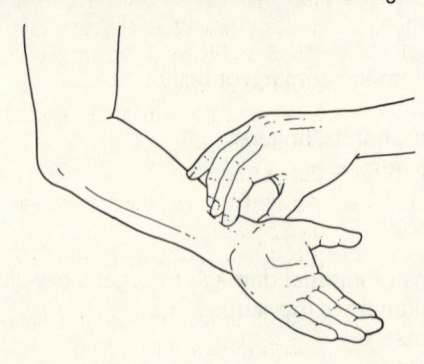

3. Press very slightly. You should feel a regular beat; this is the pulse.
4. Count it for a full minute looking at your watch: the number of beats you count in one minute is the pulse rate.

Normally it is between 70 and 80 per minute.

It increases with:
- effort (so take the pulse when the patient has rested)
- fever (38°C = around 100
         39°C = around 120)
- dehydration (a pulse rate of 130 without fever may be a sign of severe dehydration)
- some diseases of the heart.

Fig. 1.2 Counting the pulse

---

smaller). If this does not happen and the pupils remain dilated (large), this usually means that they are not getting enough blood.

Normally both pupils get either bigger or smaller together. If they do not, this may mean that the brain is damaged or has some pressure on it (e.g. a blood clot). Possible causes include injury such as a broken skull, concussion (stunning), or a stroke. (But remember that it is normal for some people to have pupils of different sizes.) An overdose of certain drugs may also affect the pupils. This can be seen in people who take drugs such as morphia and heroin, which make the pupils of the eye very small indeed (pin-point).

PAIN

A conscious patient is likely to tell you when he has

pain. Asking him questions and making observations in an orderly manner will give you vital information about that pain. For example:

Ask: Where does it hurt?
Then note: The general body area which the patient indicates; e.g. arm.
The specific body structure indicated; e.g. the elbow.
Extent of painful area; e.g. above or below the elbow.

Ask: What kind of pain?
Then note: Whether it is a sharp pain, or
a dull pain, or
a radiating pain (one which spreads), or
a slight or tolerable pain (one which is bearable and not 'too bad'), or
a severe and intolerable pain (one which needs medicine to take it away).

Ask: When does it hurt?
Then note: Whether it is all the time, or
now and again (it comes and goes), or
only when that part of the body is touched, or
only when part of the body is moved.

Ask: How long has it hurt?
Then note: Whether it is since injury, or
has been hurting for a day, or hours or minutes, or
whether it came on slowly (gradual onset), or
whether it came on quickly (sudden onset).

If the patient is frightened, the pain may feel worse.

In some instances of shock, mental illness, or when drugs or alcohol have been taken, pain may not be felt acutely.

Absence of pain does not mean that there is no serious injury. If nerves are damaged, pain from even severe injuries may not be felt by the patient.

ABILITY TO MOVE

Normal movements of the body depend upon normal functioning (working) of the body.

Paralysis can mean that there is damage to nerves, the spinal cord or to the brain.

If movement is slight or painful, it may mean that there is injury to the muscles and bones.

**Extreme care must be exercised when examining a patient to find out whether he can move parts of his body.**

**If the spinal cord is broken or injured, movement can cause severe and serious damage—even paralysis of both legs and both arms.**

**The patient should never be asked to show you how much he can move unless you are sure that the movement will not cause further injury.**

NUMBNESS

A loss of feeling when touched (numbness) may be because of damage to nerves or to the blood supply to that part of the body.

SWELLING

A collection of blood or other body fluids will produce swelling. This shows more in tissues (flesh and skin) which are close to the surface of the body. Swelling may be caused by injury, infection, an allergy (sensitivity to something) or from a fault in the circulation of the blood.

DEFORMITY (APPEARANCE OR POSITIONING OF PART OF THE BODY WHICH IS NOT NORMAL)

Injury to a part of the body may produce an abnormal positioning or appearance of that part. Dislocated (out of place) joints and some fractures (broken bones) produce deformity. How great this is can be seen by comparing the injured side with the corresponding uninjured side.

DISCHARGE FROM OPENINGS IN THE BODY (ORIFICES)

Blood, mucus or other fluid coming from any opening of the body when you cannot see any injury usually means internal (inside) injuries. You should note the colour, the consistency (e.g. watery, jelly-like) and the amount of any discharge (see also page 45).

FEELING AND BEING SICK (NAUSEA AND VOMITING)

Feeling sick (nausea) or being sick (vomiting) or both, can mean that the belly (stomach and gut) is poisoned or infected. Being or feeling sick can also be caused by stress, injury or other illnesses. You should notice the amount, colour and consistency of any vomit. This information could help you and others to decide what is wrong with the ill person.

## FITS (CONVULSIONS)

A very high body temperature, a condition called epilepsy, brain disease or damage, and certain poisons, e.g. paraquat, can cause fits. Your main responsibility is to see that the patient is able to breathe and does no injury to himself. You should also notice how deep the fits are (level of consciousness: see page 4) and how long they last (see also page 29).

The signs and symptoms given here are the major clues you will need to help you to decide the emergency with which you are dealing, and what first aid you should give. You will find them if you observe (look carefully), listen and palpate (feel). Finding such clues depends not upon shiny instruments, but upon using your own five senses. Possible meanings of these important clues, and also of some other signs and symptoms, are given throughout this book.

## 3. Giving the appropriate first aid

Choosing the right first aid depends upon your interpretation of all the information you have collected.

Treatment of those conditions which are a threat to life must be given before you look for other injuries.

Once the most serious conditions have been taken care of, then you can continue with further examination of the patient.

The stopping of breathing and heart pumping (cardio-pulmonary arrest) and profuse bleeding are given the highest priority. Quickness is vital if life is to be *saved*. You must act at once when either of these happens.

Poisoning and severe shock must be treated next.

Then deal with the emergencies which require immediate treatment if life is to be *maintained*. These include coma (when you cannot wake the patient), heart attack, stroke, large burns, heat stroke and internal bleeding.

Difficult childbirth, or problems during childbirth, should also be considered as emergencies to which you must give speedy attention.

When treating someone who has been badly injured there are eleven points to remember:

(1) Treat the patient on the spot, unless it is dangerous to do so (e.g. he is in a blazing house).
(2) Maintain a clear airway for him (see page 10).
(3) Control any bleeding (see page 17).
(4) Treat for shock.
(5) Be very aware that while carrying out emergency treatment you can cause further injury. This is particularly so when caring for patients with injuries to the head, neck and spine. Wrong handling can lead to disability or even death (see page 5).
(6) Calm the injured person and give him confidence that you know what you are doing.
(7) Cover any open wounds (see page 21).
(8) Do not try to push back any bone which is sticking out.
(9) Prevent the patient from moving any broken bones.
(10) Keep the patient as comfortable as is possible.
(11) Continue to watch the patient's condition (and to act as this may indicate), until you have him at the hospital or health centre.

Injuries to muscle and bone are generally not a threat to life, but even minor injuries can be dangerous. Proper care can prevent permanent damage and disability.

### Shock

Shock is a condition which can quickly cause death. It is caused by a severe drop in the patient's blood pressure. This may be due to loss of blood, severe, continuous pain, a large burn, severe illness, dehydration (lack of sufficient water in the body), or severe allergic reaction (sensitive response to something). Sometimes you may not be able to see the loss of fluid (e.g. into a crushed limb or from other internal bleeding), but in these instances fluid is lost rapidly from the patient's general circulation, because it goes into the body tissues and stays there.

SIGNS AND SYMPTOMS

- The patient becomes pale and cold.
- His skin will be moist and clammy.
- Sweat will appear on his forehead.
- The pulse will be weak and fast.
- Breathing will become rapid and shallow.
- There may be vomiting or a feeling of sickness.
- His mouth will be dry.
- He may lose consciousness.
- If conscious, the patient will probably say that he feels very weak and thirsty.

TREATMENT

Arrangements should be made for transport to a health centre or hospital as soon as possible. If this is

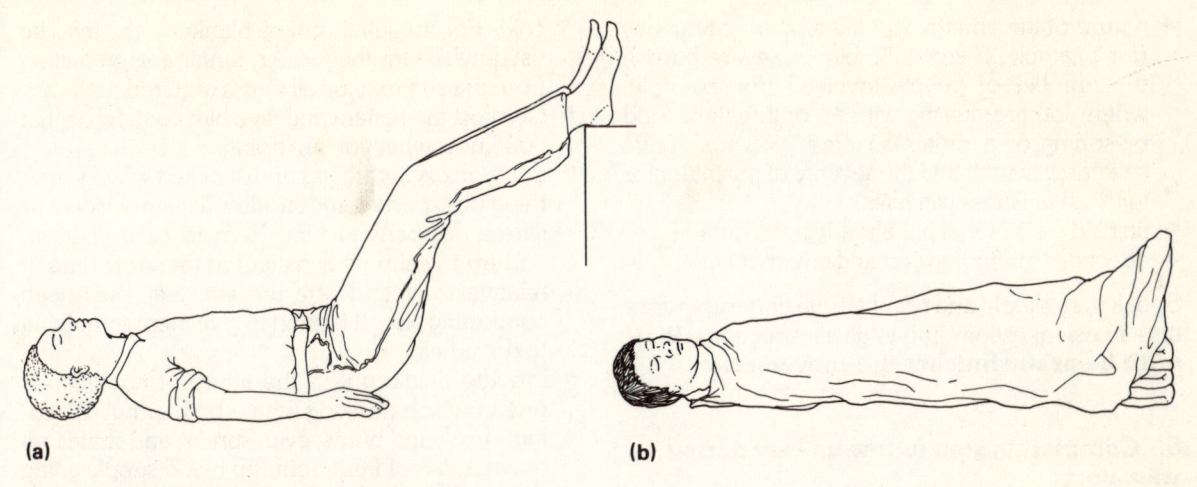

*Fig. 1.3 Positions for the treatment of shock*

not possible, seek advice from your supervisor. In the meantime:

- Lie the patient flat, with the head and body level but the legs raised a little to help the blood to return to the heart (Fig. 1.3a). (The whole body should *not* be tipped: this could result in a reduction of blood returning from the head and cause swelling of the brain. It could also cause internal organs to hinder breathing.)
- If the patient is cold, cover them with blankets, coats or any warm material to hand (Fig. 1.3b).
- If he is conscious, give him warm fluids to drink.
- If he is in pain, give aspirin.
- Keep calm, and reassure the patient.
- If consciousness is lost, maintain the patient's airway (see page 10).
- If there is bleeding, deal with that quickly (see page 17).
- If there is vomiting, the patient should be put into a position which prevents him from breathing in the vomit (see page 10 and Fig. 2.6).
- All movements should be carried out with great care, especially if a brain or spinal injury is suspected (see page 5).
- The patient should be protected from extreme heat and cold.
- Fluids lost must be replaced as quickly and as soon as possible—intravenously if necessary, and if you or someone else who is present knows how to do this.

Everyone who gives first aid must be aware of the possibility of shock developing in all injured or dehydrated people. Quick action in the early stages can prevent further development which can lead to death.

Once the injuries or conditions which are threatening your patient's life have been controlled, your examination of him must be continued. Only in this way can you be sure you do not miss another injury or condition which also requires treatment.

## 4. Notifying your supervisor and arranging transport

By its very meaning, first aid is temporary and immediate treatment only. All emergencies you have treated should be seen later by your supervisor. Send patients to the nearest health centre or hospital as soon as you have done what you can to save or maintain life at the place the emergency happens, and after you have obtained transport for the journey.

As you *begin* giving first aid, tell anyone present to call for assistance, to send for transport or make something on which to carry the patient (e.g. improvise a stretcher from bamboo and coats or banana leaves).

Certain information must be given to your supervisor when you contact him or her for advice or transport. It is important to think through a sequence in which you are going to give this information, in order to make sure that nothing of importance is left out. Give the following information always:

- indentification: your own name and the name of the place where you are;

- nature of the emergency: the type of emergency (for example, a crocodile bite or severe burns); the number of people involved (for example, when you are dealing with an outbreak of food poisoning or a motor-car crash you may have several patients), and the severity of the injury (or injuries) or illness (illnesses);
- first aid given: what has already been done;
- directions for finding you and your patient.

Speak very clearly and calmly. Give your supervisor time to ask questions and to give instructions. **Wait until he or she finishes the conversation**.

## 5. Completing your follow-up care during transport

Treatments which support, add to or follow up the first aid given are called 'follow-up care'. Instructions for follow-up care are given to you by your supervisor, and may range from general care to one particular treatment to be carried out.

If you are unable to get help and are dependent upon your own knowledge during the journey to a health centre or hospital you should give this follow-up care:

- Keep the patient's airway open and check his vital signs. This means seeing that air can be taken into the lungs and keeping a check on his pulse, respiration rates. Act accordingly if heart or breathing stops (see pages 9–11).
- Make the patient as comfortable as possible. This may mean support in the form of putting a sling on an injured arm or placing a small pillow under his head, or giving medicine to kill pain and so on.
- Keep the patient's temperature normal. This means seeing that he is neither too hot nor too cold and is protected from extremes of heat and cold. For the latter, coats, blankets, etc. may be used, whilst for the former, fanning or protection from the sun may be all that is required.
- Comfort the patient and give him confidence that you know what you are doing.
- Everyone is frightened and shocked when something unexpected and sudden, like an accident or illness, happens to him. Remain calm yourself, and try to calm your patient at the same time. If relatives or friends are present, they may need comforting also. It is good to give them something to do to help.
- Provide fluids, unless the injury or condition is one in which drinking would be harmful. Bleeding, shock and burns, even sprains and strains, all mean a loss of fluid from the blood supply going round the body. It helps to replace this as soon as possible. However, sometimes this could do harm. When, and in which conditions, this is so, is described in subsequent chapters.
- Control people standing around. This can be difficult; but injured or ill people need air and quiet, and crowds should be kept away. Tell one or two people you know are sensible to do this for you. Use other people to help you to get assistance, to improvise stretchers and even to give first aid if you have two or more patients to look after. But you must tell these helpers clearly and calmly what they should do and how they should do it.
- Complete arrangements for transport to hospital or health centre. Give your report quickly, quietly and cover all points. Carry out any further instructions you may receive.

The general procedures outlined in this chapter are intended to serve as a guide for all emergency situations. They should be borne in mind during study and practice of the remainder of the text.

# 2. What to Do when Someone Cannot Breathe Properly

## Respiratory (breathing) and cardiac (heart) emergencies

Breathing is essential to life. In all cases where the patient is unconscious, or has a serious injury, even if there are other more obvious injuries, you must first check that his airway is clear and that his breathing is adequate to maintain life. Check his pulse at the same time.

If there is any breathing (respiratory) difficulty, make particular note of the following:

(1) respiration: the rate and depth of breathing and whether it is regular (even) or irregular (uneven);
(2) heart rate: do this by taking the pulse: note its power (volume) and whether it is regular (even) or irregular (uneven);
(3) skin: the colour of palms, soles, eyelids: its temperature: whether it feels cool and moist when touched.

Loosen any tight clothing around the patient's neck and waist so that his chest movements are not limited by them.

## Stoppage of breathing (respiratory arrest)

Breathing will stop if the airway (nose, throat and windpipe to the lungs) becomes blocked, compressed or narrowed. Urgent treatment is necessary when this happens. It is the most serious complication of some respiratory diseases, of severe shock, or of injury. The treatment is to put air into the patient's lungs for him until they begin to work again.

## Conditions which may lead to respiratory arrest

The following may result in respiratory arrest:

- Severe spasm (contraction) of the windpipe (trachea or bronchus).
  Causes include inhalation of a small amount of food, water, smoke or irritant gas; hiccups; bronchitis; and asthma.

- Obstruction of the airway.
  The cause of this may be the tongue falling back into the throat. This may happen when an unconscious patient is left lying on his back. Other causes include swelling of the inside of the throat because of an allergy, insect stings, or burns from swallowing corrosives (some kinds of chemicals), or the breathing in of a piece of food or loosened tooth (e.g. during a fight when the mouth is hit).

- Suffocation (smothering).
  This may be due to a piece of material, a pillow or a plastic bag, etc. completely covering the nose and mouth.

- Compression of the neck.
  This is caused by strangulation or by hanging.

- Compression of the chest.
  This can be caused by a fall of earth, sand or grain in a silo; crushing against a hard object; a penetrating wound or the kind of chest injury often seen in a road-traffic accident.

- Damage to the nerves controlling breathing.
  This can be caused by electrocution; animal, insect or reptile bites; muscle spasm from tetanus (an infection caused by certain germs— see page 23), poisoning or paralysis (e.g. poliomyelitis).
  Sometimes the amount of oxygen in the air is not adequate. This happens when poisonous gases are present (e.g. exhaust fumes from a motor-car) or at very high altitudes or during deep-sea diving. Another cause can be continuous fits (see page 62).

## Signs and symptoms

- Loss of consciousness (sometimes sudden collapse).

## First Aid

- No visible breathing (sometimes gasping on and off).
- Blueness of lips and inside of mouth.
- General pallor (paleness)—including soles of feet and palms of hands (in dark-skinned people).

Unless artificial respiration (breathing for the patient) is begun immediately, the heart will be starved of oxygen and will cease to beat. That means death.

### Treatment

- Shout for help.
- Whilst doing so, ensure that the patient's airway is clear. To do this, place the patient flat on his back with the head turned to one side (Fig. 2.1). Remove anything which is preventing the taking-in of air (i.e. plastic bag over head, or rope around the neck, etc.). Scoop out with your fingers, which you have wrapped in a piece of soft cloth, any vomit, loose teeth etc. in the mouth (Fig. 2.2).
- Kneel beside the patient's head. Place one hand under his neck and the other hand under his lower jaw. Extend his head and neck gently backwards (Fig. 2.3). This prevents the tongue from falling back into the throat.
- Take a very deep breath and hold it.
- Fit your mouth tightly over the patient's open mouth and forcibly breathe out into his lungs (Fig. 2.4). Keep one of your hands supporting his neck, but use the other to gently pinch his nostrils together as you breathe into his mouth. The air will be expelled from the patient without help.

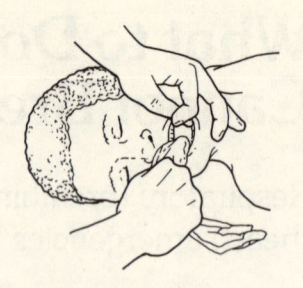

*Fig. 2.2 Cleaning out the patient's mouth*

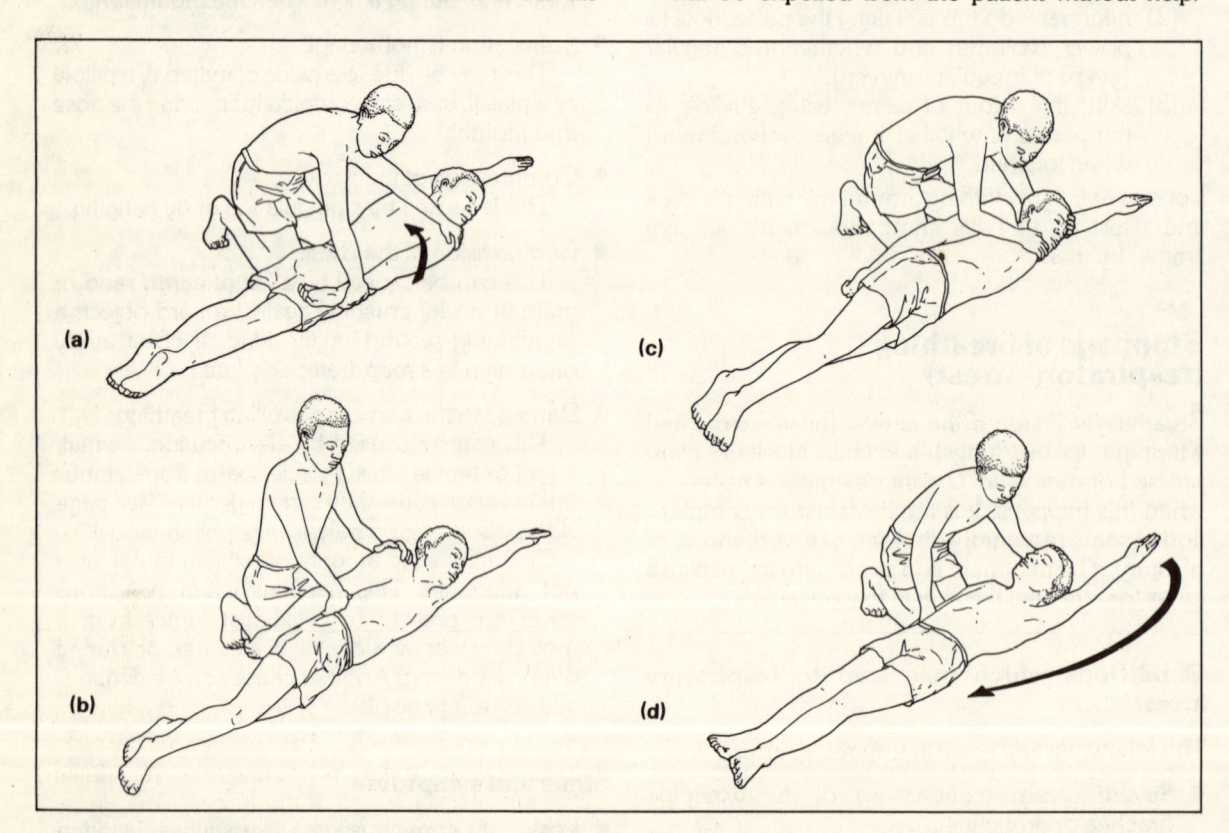

*Fig. 2.1 Turning the patient on to his back*

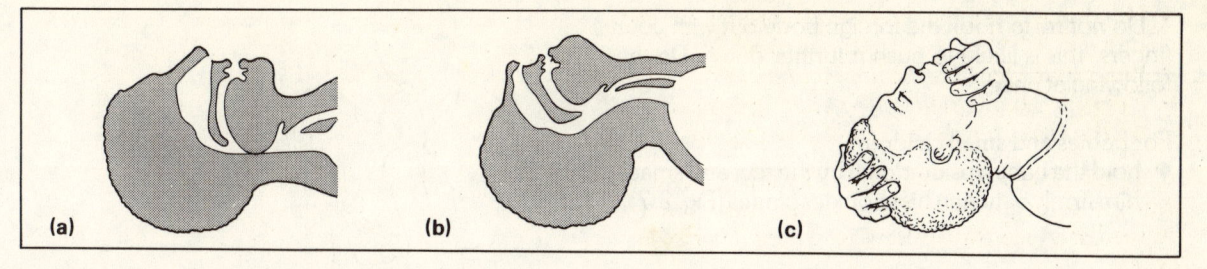

*Fig. 2.3 Airway (a) blocked by the tongue, and (b) cleared by extending patient's head and neck; (c) external view*

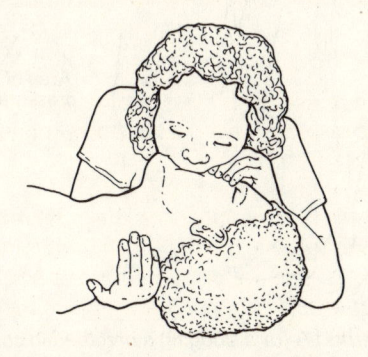

*Fig. 2.4 Mouth to mouth artificial respiration*

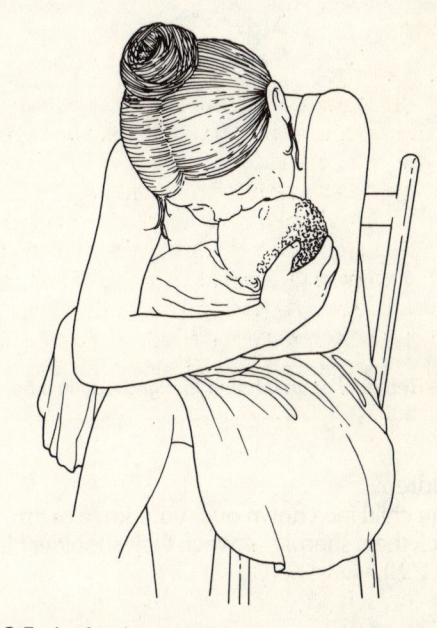

*Fig. 2.5 Artificial respiration of a young child or baby showing the mouth-to-mouth-and-nose position*

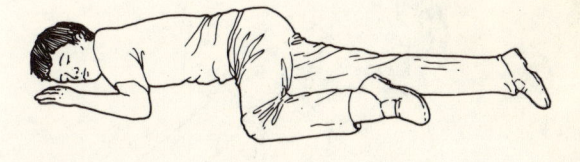

*Fig. 2.6 The recovery position*

You should observe during this procedure whether his chest rises and falls. If it does not, either there is an air-leak around the mouth and your mouth is not positioned firmly or tightly enough, or the patient's airway is blocked. In the latter case, repeat the procedure for clearing his mouth and extend his neck again before continuing.

- Whilst carrying out artificial respiration, check the patient's pulse every 2 or 3 minutes to ensure that the heart has not stopped (cardiac arrest).
- Continue the breathing procedure at a rate of 12 to 18 breaths per minute until the chest is seen to rise and the patient is breathing for himself, or until you are certain he is dead. (You may have to keep up the procedure for an hour or more).

If the patient is a child, both his nose and mouth should be covered by your mouth. Very gentle breathing—short puffs—should be used and the younger the child, the more gentle this should be (Fig. 2.5). Continue at a rate of 25 breaths per minute.

Once the patient can breathe by himself, place him in what is called 'the recovery position' (Fig. 2.6). Even if he appears perfectly alright, inform your supervisor of what has happened. Something could go wrong later.

## Choking

A small piece of food or a bone (in this instance it is called a foreign body), may be inhaled into the windpipe when eating. Most people on such occasions are able to cough it up at once. Sometimes, however, this may not be possible and help is needed.

12   First Aid

Do *not* try to hook the foreign body out with your fingers: this is likely to push it further down. Do the following at once:

For babies and small children:
- hold the baby upside-down by the feet and smack him firmly between his shoulder blades (Fig. 2.7).

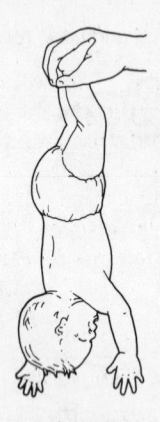

*Fig. 2.7 Removal of an inhaled foreign body in a baby*

For children:
- lie the child face down over your knee or arm and smack them sharply between their shoulder blades (Fig. 2.8).

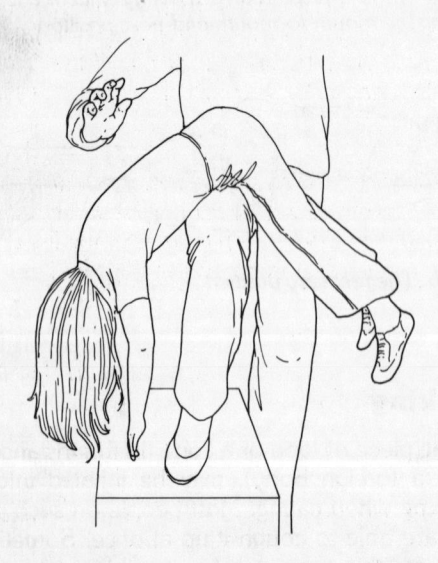

*Fig. 2.8 Removal of an inhaled foreign body in a child*

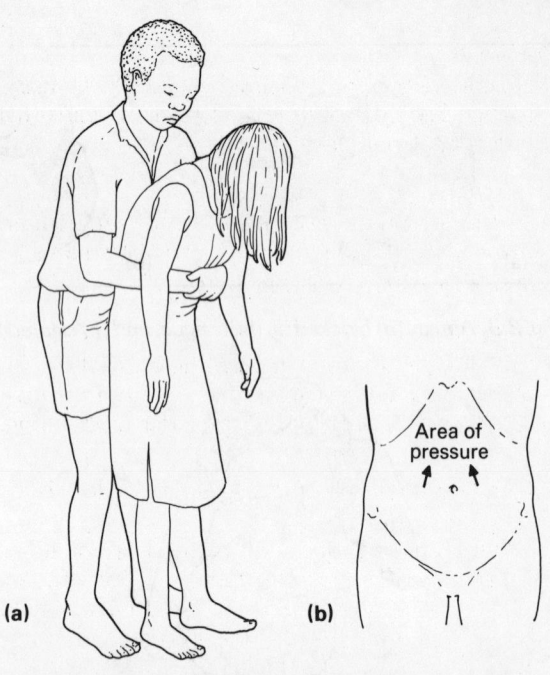

*Fig. 2.9 Method A for dislodging a breathed in chunk of food showing (a) the important positioning of the first aider's hands and (b) the area of pressure on the patient*

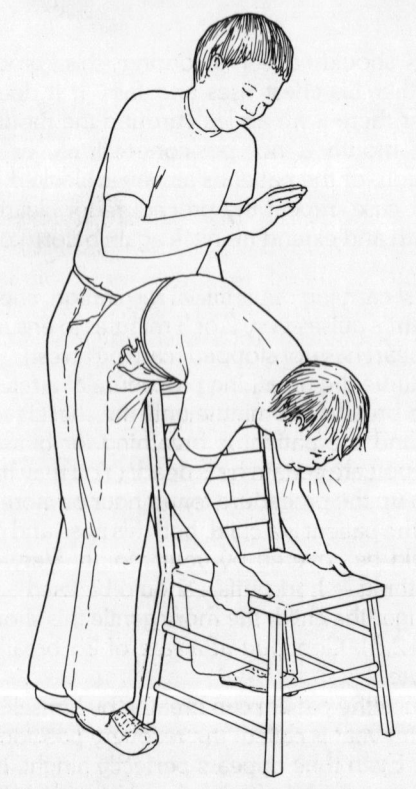

*Fig. 2.10 Method B for dislodging breathed in chunk of food*

For adults:
- There are two methods and either may be used, depending upon the circumstances and your own knowledge and practice.

*Method A:*
- Stand behind the patient and grasp them around the chest just under the chest bone (sternum).

Give a short sharp bear hug. (Fig. 2.9).

*Method B:*
- Tell the patient to lean over the back of a chair holding on to the seat and then bang him sharply 3 or 4 times between his shoulder blades. (Fig. 2.10).

Whichever method you use, the foreign body should be coughed out.

When very soft food, drink, blood or vomit has been breathed in, place the patient in the recovery position (Fig. 2.6), and clear his mouth of any food or vomit with your fingers (wrapped in a soft, clean cloth). If breathing has stopped, begin mouth-to-mouth respiration.

## Drowning

Drowning can happen in many different places: sea, river, lake, swamp, spring, bath and so on.

You should begin artificial respiration at once. Do not wait to get water out of the patient's chest first. Do clear his mouth of any seaweed etc. If you cannot get air into his lungs, quickly turn the patient on his side, putting his head lower than his legs and push his body (just under the chest bone) with the heel (the part between wrist and palm) of your hand. Then give mouth-to-mouth respiration.

## Acute attack of asthma

Asthma can be a chronic (life-long) disease, but a person who has this illness may have acute attacks from time to time.

This means that he has great difficulty in breathing and will make a hissing or wheezing sound, especially when breathing out. You may see that the skin behind his collar bone and between his ribs gets sucked in when he tries to take a breath. Although asthma may be a problem throughout life, it is generally worse during certain months of the year and at night time.

An acute attack may be brought on by eating or breathing in something to which the patient is allergic. A number of children who suffer from asthma sometimes have an acute attack when they have a head cold.

If asthma is worse when inside the house, the patient should go outside where the air is cleaner or to an open window. You should remain calm, quiet and gentle and give reassurance (comfort and confidence) to the patient. Find him the most comfortable position: this is likely to be leaning forward with his elbows resting on a table so that his lungs are stretched. Give him warm liquids in sips. Sometimes breathing steam helps to loosen mucus and so help breathing. See that the patient has something into which he can spit out sputum (coughed up matter).

For mild attacks of asthma, ephedrine or theophylline are sometimes given. If the attack is severe, adrenaline is usually injected. If the attack is prolonged, contact your supervisor and obtain advice or assistance.

## Heart (cardiac) emergencies

As breathing is essential to life, so is the ability of the heart to circulate blood around the body. Any loss or decrease in this pumping action can lead to disablement, while total failure means death.

You should make the same observations of patients suffering from heart emergencies as those listed for breathing emergencies (page 9), as the two systems are very closely linked.

In heart and breathing illnesses or damage, the circulation to more distant parts of the body is very often poor. This means that you may not be able to feel pulses near the feet and hands. If this is so, feel for pulses nearer to the heart. The three methods of doing this are:

- Palpating (feeling) the carotid pulse in the neck. This is easily found by turning the patient's head a little to the side and moving your fingers directly down from the lobe of his ear (Fig. 2.11).

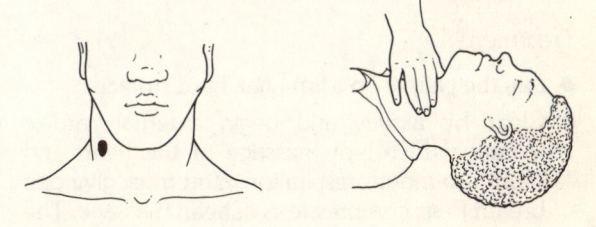

*Fig. 2.11 The position (a) and palpatation (b) of the neck (carotid) pulse*

14  First Aid

- Palpating the femoral pulse in his groin (inside of the top of the thigh) (Fig. 2.12).

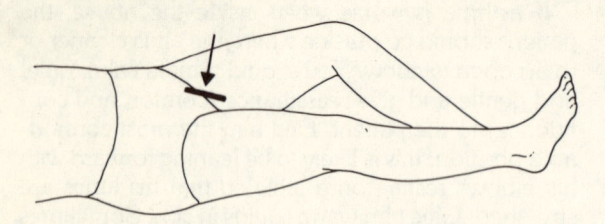

*Fig. 2.12 The position of the leg (femoral) pulse*

- Listening to the apex beat of his heart by placing your ear on the patient's chest just below his left nipple.

## Cardiac arrest (the heart has stopped)

*Signs and symptoms*

- Unconsciousness; often a sudden collapse.
- No pulse can be felt.
- There is no sign of breathing.
- The pupils are dilating (becoming larger than normal) or, if 40 seconds or more after collapse, pupils are already dilated.
- The skin changes colour: it becomes paler or blue.

The patient is, in effect, dead.

**If he has been like this for 3 minutes or more** DO NOTHING.

If the collapse happens whilst you are there and **if you act within 3 minutes**, you can try to prevent death. If other people are within hearing, shout for help, as you prepare to treat the patient.

*Treatment*

- Lay the patient on a firm, flat, hard surface.
- Clear his airway and begin external cardiac massage (ECM) or massage of the heart and mouth-to-mouth respiration. You must give one breath to six compressions of heart massage. The patient's lungs should be filled with air before you begin the heart massage.

## External cardiac massage (ECM)

The aim of heart massage is to press the heart between the breast bone (sternum) and the back bone (spine), thus literally squeezing blood out of it (Fig. 2.13).

- Lie the patient on a firm flat surface. Kneel close to his side, at right angles to him and alongside his chest. Press the lower third of his breast bone sharply with the heels of your hands (the heel is the part between the wrist and palm), using pressure from your *shoulders* (Fig. 2.14). Do not bend

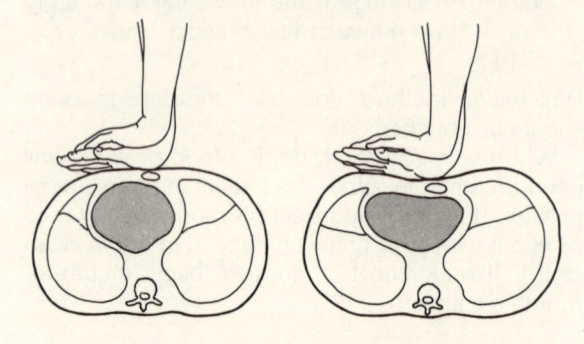

*Fig. 2.13 Pressing the heart between the breast bone and the spine*

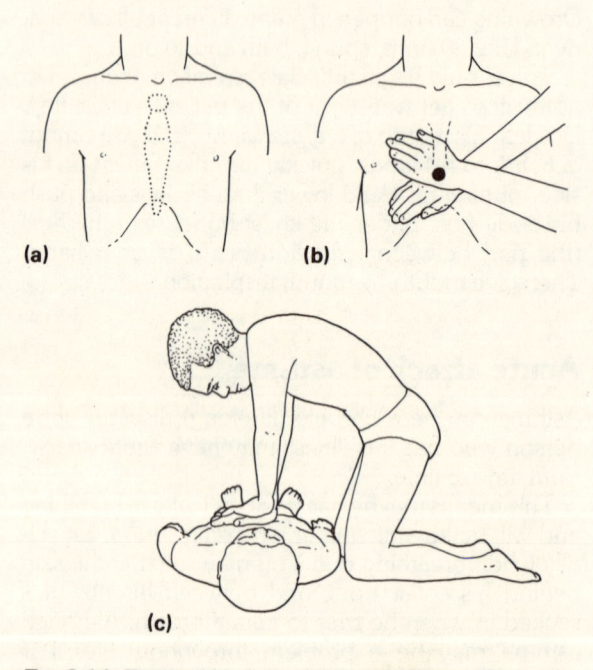

*Fig. 2.14 External cardiac massage: (a) the position of the sternum showing the area (shaded) to be compressed; (b) the heels of the hands on the lower third of the sternum and (c) the straight arms working from the shoulders*

# Respiratory and Cardiac Emergencies

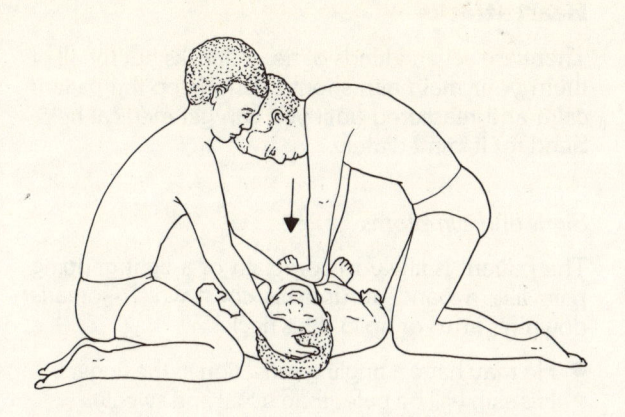

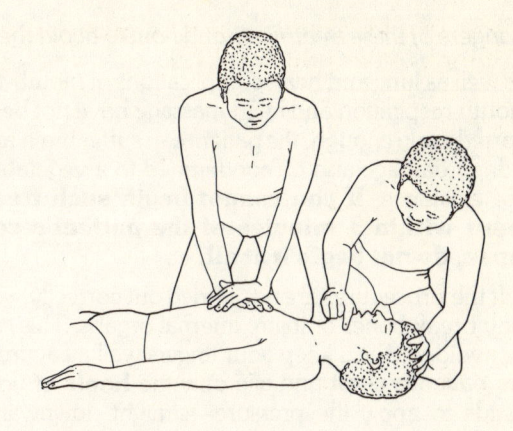

*Fig. 2.15 External cardiac massage on an adult with two operators showing alternative positions*

your arms at the elbows. The rate of these compressions (or pressures) should be 70–80 per minute (the normal pulse rate).
- Check the carotid pulse (see page 13) every few minutes to see if the heart beat has re-started.
- If you are succeeding, the pupils of your patient's eyes will begin to get smaller. Check these from time to time.

Although it is possible for one person to carry out both artificial respiration and ECM, it is very tiring and if possible two of you should work together. One should see that the airway is clear, carry out the mouth-to-mouth respiration, and check the pulse and pupils, whilst the other peforms ECM (Fig. 2.15). There should be a short pause after every sixth heart massage to allow the patient's lungs to fill with air. Do not forget to check that the patient's chest is moving: it should rise and fall with each respiration.

Cardiac massage and mouth-to-mouth respiration can be continued by two people for a considerable time if they change places every few minutes.

If the patient's pulse returns, check whether breathing has also begun: it may be necessary to continue the artificial respiration without the massage.

Once the heart is beating and the patient is breathing, the patient should be placed in the recovery position (Fig. 2.6). Contact your supervisor for further advice. Continue to note the pulse and respirations. Even if the person recovers and appears to be alright, he must be seen in a health centre or hospital. Something could go wrong later.

## Heart massage for babies and children

The younger the child, the less pressure you should use when compressing the lower third of the breast bone (sternum). In children, enough pressure is obtained by using the heel of only one hand (Fig. 2.16) and for babies use only two fingers (Fig. 2.17).

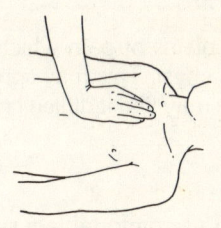

*Fig. 2.16 External cardiac massage on a child*

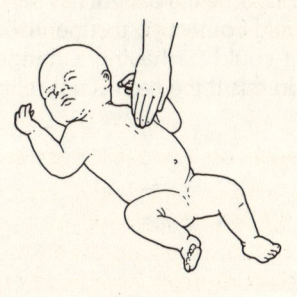

*Fig. 2.17 External cardiac massage on a baby*

*Dangers of these treatments and how to avoid them*

As well as lung and heart complications, if mouth-to-mouth respiration and heart massage have not been started early enough, the patient can suffer brain and kidney damage and be condemned to a vegetable-like existence. **If you cannot begin such treatment within 3 minutes of the patient's collapse, do not begin it at all.**

If the procedures are not carried out correctly, you may break bones or injure internal organs. This can be avoided if you keep your fingers well away from the patient's chest and use only the **heels** of your hands to apply the pressure—straight downwards from your shoulders with elbows kept straight. Pressure should only be applied to the lower one-third of the breast bone and never to elsewhere on the chest.

## Angina

When the blood supply to the heart is reduced because of disease, the patient may experience some pain when he takes exercise, when he is worried, or after he has eaten a big meal. This is likely to be a condition called angina.

*Signs and symptoms*

The patient complains of pain which is like a tight band around his chest. This may spread down one or both arms. He may find it difficult to breathe.

*Treatment*

Sit the patient in as comfortable a position as possible. If the condition has already been diagnosed by a doctor, he is likely to have glycerine trinitrate pills (TNT) to place under the patient's tongue. Give him one. Pain will usually pass within a few minutes.

If this is the fist time the patient has had this kind of pain, you should contact your supervisor for advice as the patient could be having a dangerous heart attack. Also do this if the pain is not relieved by the TNT.

## Heart attacks

There are several kinds of heart attacks but for all of them your main aim should be to keep the patient calm and reassured until you can get medical help. Send for it immediately.

*Signs and symptoms*

The patient is likely to complain of a tight gripping pain like a band around his chest which spreads down his arms or up into his neck.

- He may have a tingling sensation in the fingers.
- His skin will be paler than usual and sweaty.
- There will be difficulty in breathing.
- His pulse will be weak and rapid.
- He may vomit.

*Treatment*

Help the patient to a comfortable position: this is usually one which is called the semi-recumbent position (Fig. 2.18).

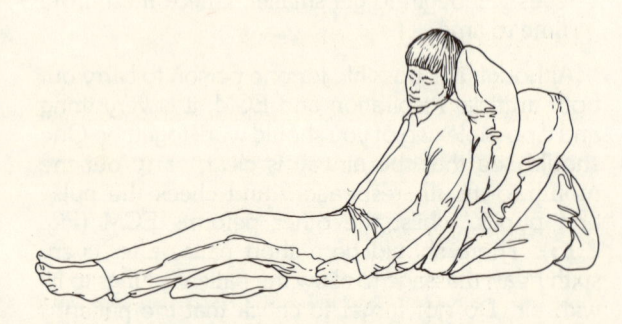

*Fig. 2.18 The semi-recumbent position*

- Sips of water may be taken, but no alcohol.
- Contact your supervisor for advice regarding long-term care.

# 3. What to Do when Someone has a Bad Cut or Wound

A wound is cut or torn skin and flesh or other body tissues. It may be internal (inside) or external (outside). Your main aims when dealing with a wound are:

(1) to control the bleeding (haemorrhage);
(2) to treat shock;
(3) to maintain function (help the patient to breathe and blood to circulate);
(4) to prevent complications (particularly by reducing the risk of infection).

## Bleeding and its control

Types of bleeding from a wound are grouped according to the type of blood vessels damaged.

### Capillary bleeding

This is bleeding from the very small blood vessels called capillaries. This happens when wounds are superficial (on the surface). Blood just oozes from the cut or tear. This kind of bleeding usually stops without treatment, because nature causes clotting to take place. First aid measures may be needed, however, if the wound covers a large area: it should then be covered with clean iced water or very cold water compresses. These are made by wringing out several clean pieces of material in clean cold water or by sandwiching ice between layers of clean material.

### Venous bleeding

Venous bleeding is bleeding from veins. Dark red blood flows from the wound. If large veins are involved this loss can be brisk, and is then a threat to life. To stop this bleeding you should raise the bleeding part above the rest of the patient's body. (If this is a leg or arm, elevating it will, in the first place, increase the flow of blood because venous blood flows towards the heart, but it will lessen in a short time.)

### Arterial bleeding

Arterial bleeding is bleeding from an artery. The blood is bright red and spurts from the wound. People can quickly bleed to death when an artery is cut. Controlling this bleeding takes second place **only** to treating cardiac or respiratory arrest.

There are basically three methods for controlling bleeding and they should be used in the following order:

(1) *Direct pressure*

Hard, direct pressure applied directly over the wound controls bleeding in most cases (Fig. 3.1).

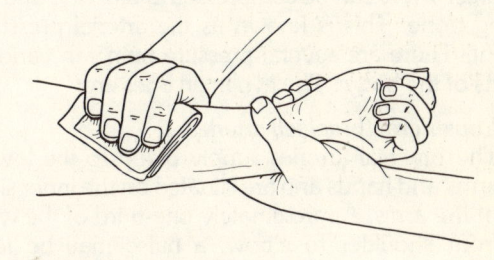

*Fig. 3.1 Direct pressure over a wound*

The pressure should be continued until a clean, firm-pressure (very thick) dressing can be applied (Fig. 3.2).

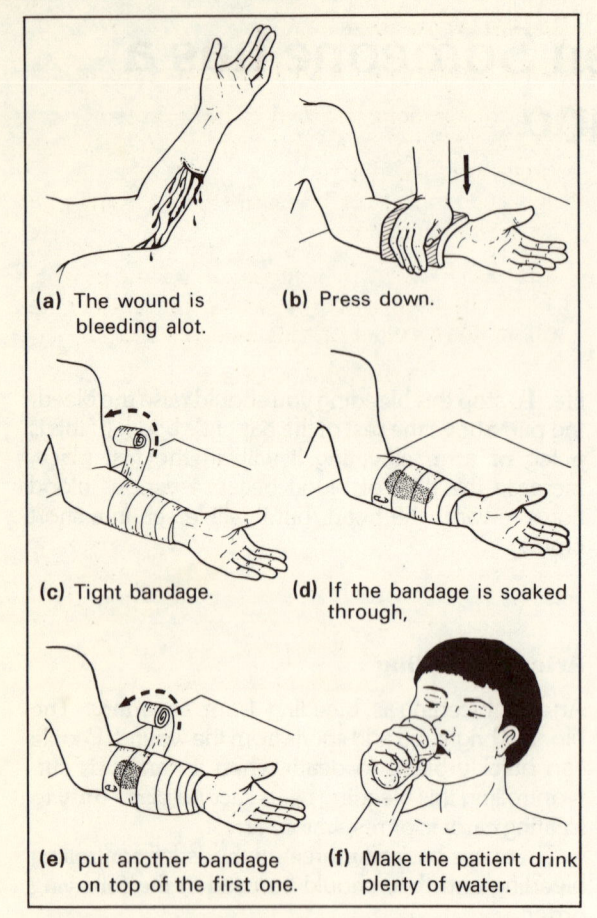

*Fig. 3.2 a–f. Applying pressure and a thick dressing to a wound*

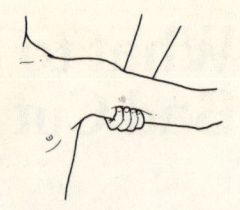

(a) The wound is bleeding alot.
(b) Press down.
(c) Tight bandage.
(d) If the bandage is soaked through,
(e) put another bandage on top of the first one.
(f) Make the patient drink plenty of water.

*Fig. 3.3 Application of pressure to the arm (brachial) pulse*

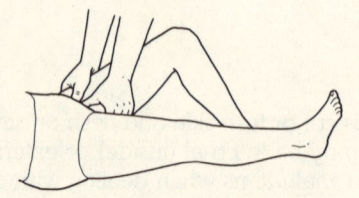

*Fig. 3.4 Application of pressure to the leg (femoral) pulse*

### (2) Arterial pressure

Should direct pressure not control the bleeding, pressure can be applied to the point at which the nearest artery can be compressed against the underlying bone. This is known as the arterial pressure point. There are several pressure points in various parts of the body. The two main ones are:

I  *Lower arm (brachial) arteries*
   The brachial arteries supply blood to the lower arms and hands and are situated on the inner side of the arms. Approximately one-third of the way from shoulder to elbow, a pulse may be felt. Pressure should be applied to that point (Fig. 3.3).
II *Leg (femoral) arteries*
   Pulses from the femoral arteries can be felt in the groins (Fig. 3.4). Bleeding from these arteries can be very severe and you should learn to locate and apply pressure to the pulses rapidly.

In cases of very severe bleeding, manual pressure over the main artery nearest to the bleeding point should be applied **as well** as direct pressure over the wound itself.

This method of stopping bleeding is limited by the difficulty of keeping up the pressure for any length of time, and particularly when moving and transporting the patient.

When you apply a pressure dressing (Fig. 3.5) to a limb, use folded cloth or a wide belt. Never use thin rope, string or wire. Loosen the tie every 20 minutes to see whether it is still needed. Leaving it on too long can damage a leg or arm so badly that it has to be cut off.

## Local cures

There are some plant juices (e.g. cardon, cactus juice) which help to stop superficial bleeding. If local ones are good, cut a stalk with a clean knife and apply it firmly against the wound. When the bleeding is controlled, tie a piece of the cactus to the wound with a bit of clean cloth. After 2 or 3 hours, take off the stalk and clean the wound with boiled water.

Never use lime, coffee, tea, kerosene, dung or dirt to stop bleeding.

## Care of wounds

### Surface (minor) wounds

Minor wounds are those which involve only the superficial layers of the skin. These should be cleaned with clean boiled water, taking care to remove all dirt. Wash your own hands very well before

# A Bad Cut or Wound 19

If the bleeding cannot be controlled by pressing on the wound, and if the person is losing alot of blood, do the following:

Keep pressing on the wound.

Keep the wounded part as high as possible.

Tie the arm or leg as close to the wound as possible — between the wound and the body. Tighten enough to control the bleeding.

For the tie, use a folded cloth or a wide belt; never use thin rope, string or wire.

*Fig. 3.5 Applying a pressure dressing to a limb*

you begin. If you have to use tweezers to remove specks of dirt or grit, boil them in water for 5 minutes before you use them. A wound may also be cleaned by putting it under a running tap if you are sure that the water supply is clean. If you have it, apply one of the commercial dressings which is already soaked with antiseptic. A freshly laundered bit of cloth (with unfolded inside surface placed next to the wound) may be used as an improvised dressing (Fig. 3.6).

Some larger surface cuts heal more quickly if they are closed or stitched.

Small wound

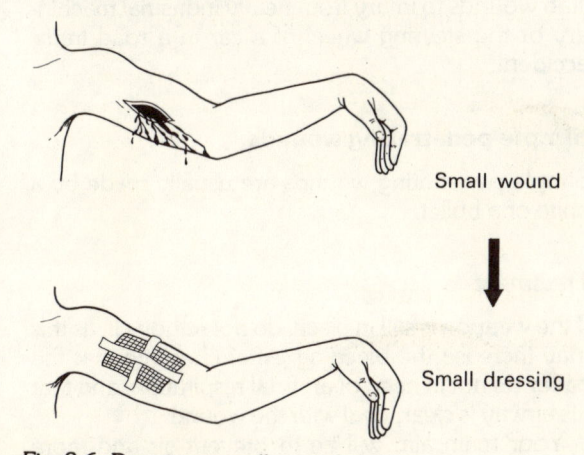

Small dressing

*Fig. 3.6 Dressing a small wound*

## Closing larger cuts

Close a deep cut only if **all** the following are true:
- the cut was done less then 12 hours ago;
- the cut is very clean and there is no dirt whatsoever hidden in it;
- it is impossible to get someone more experienced or senior to close it.

*Method I*: Butterfly sutures of adhesive tape. These are used for cuts in which the edges of the skin come together on their own (see Fig. 3.7).

How to close a wound: with sticking plaster

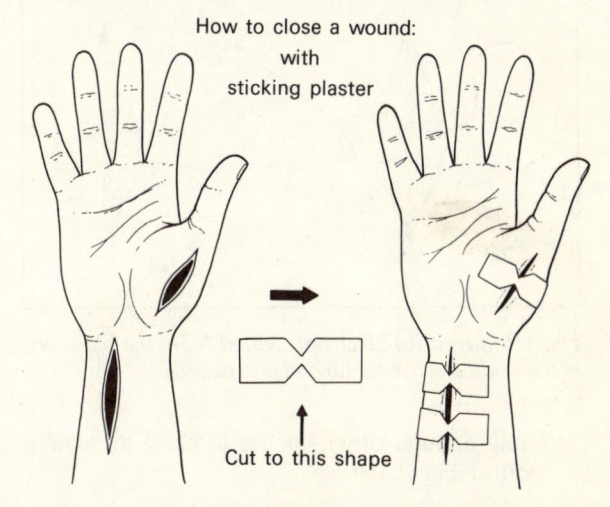

Cut to this shape

*Fig. 3.7 Closing a larger wound with sticking plaster*

*Method II*: Stitches or sutures using thread. If the edges of the skin do not come together by themselves, sutures will be required (Fig. 3.8). Again they should only be used if the wound is very clean and less than 12 hours old. Old, dirty or infected wounds must be left **open**.

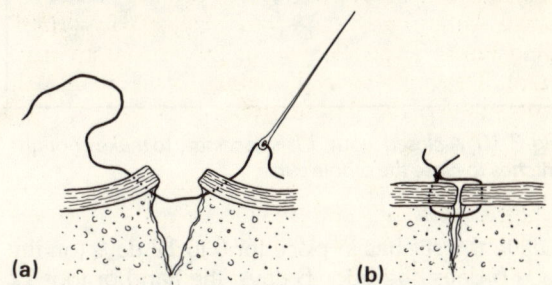

(a)  (b)

*Fig. 3.8 (a) and (b) Sutures for closing a larger wound*

Bites from dogs, pigs, people and other animals should also be left open. Closing them can cause dangerous infections, serious illnesses and even death.

## First Aid

*To stitch a wound*

- Boil a sewing needle and thin thread (nylon or silk) for 10 minutes.
- Wash the wound with clean boiled water.
- Wash your own hands very well for 3 minutes in boiled water and soap.
- Sew the wound, making the first stitch in the middle of the cut and tying it closed (Fig. 3.9).

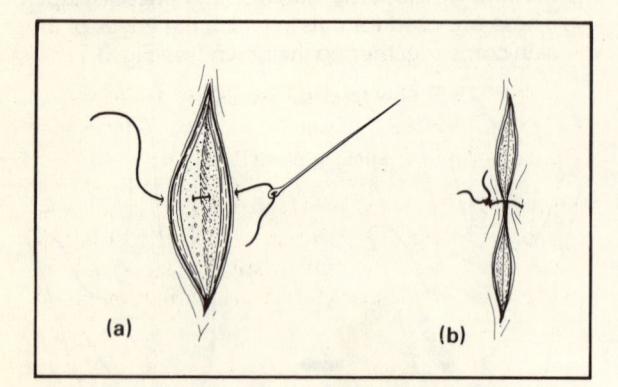

*Fig. 3.9 (a) and (b) Stitching a wound. Make the first stitch in the middle of the cut (a) and tie it closed (b).*

Make enough other stitches to close the whole wound (Fig. 3.10).

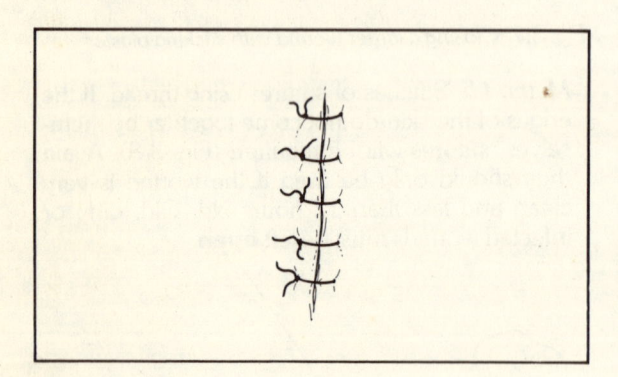

*Fig. 3.10 A closed wound. It is necessary to make enough stitches to close the whole cut.*

Leave the stitches in place for 6 to 12 days (on the face 6 days; the body 8 days; the hand or foot 12 days). Then remove the stitches: cut the thread on one side of the knot and pull the knot until the thread comes out.

**If the wound that has been closed shows any signs of infection, remove the stitches immediately and leave the wound open.**

### Major wounds

Clean the area around a major wound with clean, boiled water. If there is dirt or other foreign material in the wound this should be removed **only** if it can be done easily. **Do not probe**. Apply a clean dressing over the wound and transfer the patient to a health centre or hospital without delay. Treat for shock if necessary (page 6).

### Abdominal wounds (Belly wounds)

Abdominal wounds should be treated as major wounds and the patient treated for shock. Arrange for transport to health centre or hospital.

Internal bleeding may give little sign to begin with. If you look closely at the skin, however, you may see slight bruising over the belly. Sometimes this is the only sign of serious internal bleeding.

*Treatment*

If the contents of the belly are protruding, do **not** attempt to replace them. A sterile dressing soaked in normal saline (1 teaspoonful of salt to 1 pint of boiled water) or clean boiled water should be applied and kept moist (with more clean saline or water) until more experienced help is available:

- keep the patient flat and as still as possible;
- give no fluids by mouth;
- treat for shock, if necessary (see page 6);
- contact your supervisor for advice.

### Chest wounds

Wounds to the chest may take various forms—from stab wounds to injury from heavy industrial machinery or the steering wheel of a car in a road traffic accident.

### Simple penetrating wounds

Simple penetrating wounds are usually made by a knife or a bullet.

*Treatment*

If the weapon is still in place, do not remove it, as this may increase the bleeding. After checking that the patient is not in need of artificial respiration, and that his airway is clear, deal with the wound.

Your main aim will be to prevent air and more blood from entering the space around the lung.

Air going in through a wound can usually be heard. There will be a 'sucking' noise as the patient breathes. Dress the wound so that it is as air-tight as possible. You can do this by applying a clean dressing (sterile, if possible), covering it with a piece of polythene (or a plastic bag) and strapping it well around the edges (Fig. 3.11). A firm dressing will also help to control bleeding.

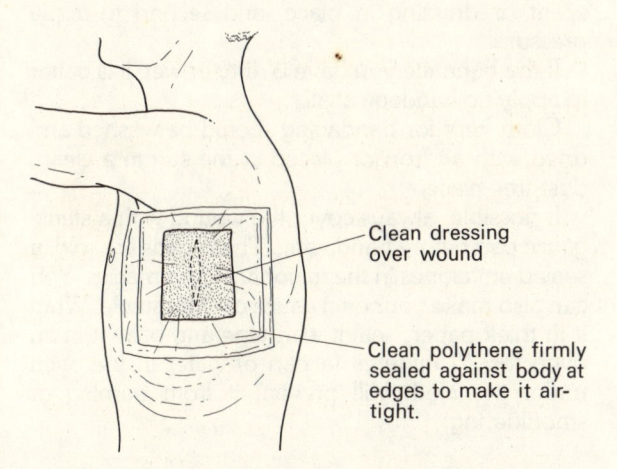

*Fig. 3.11 Strapping a chest wound when the lung is pierced*

Check for both entry and exit points of a weapon or bullet because both wounds will require dressings (Fig. 3.12).

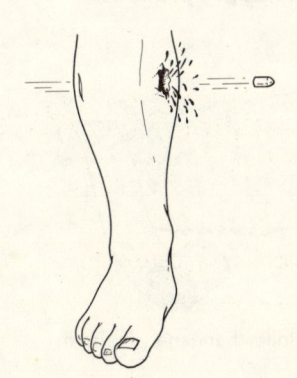

*Fig. 3.12 Gunshot wound showing the two wounds*

Treat the patient for shock, if necessary.
Give no food or drink.
Transfer the patient to a health centre or hospital as soon as possible.

## Crushed chest wounds

*Treatment*

Dress any superficial (surface) injuries.
Strap the arm on the injured side (or both arms if both sides of the chest are injured), to the patient's chest. This should be done over his clothing. While the strapping should be tight (and tightened as the patient breathes out), it should not be too tight as the end of a broken rib may be pushed against a lung and injure it.
Treat the patient for shock.
Take him to medical help as soon as possible.

## Flail Chest

Sometimes loose segments of broken ribs can cause damage to lungs and other tissues. The patient tries desperately hard to breathe, but cannot do so properly. He will be severely shocked and may cough up blood.

*Treatment*

Arrange for transfer to hospital as soon as possible.
Meanwhile, splint the chest, either by strapping a firm object such as a wodge of cloth or small pillow over the affected portion of the chest (Fig. 3.13), or by strapping the patient's arms to his chest. This splinting will help the patient to breathe on his own more easily.

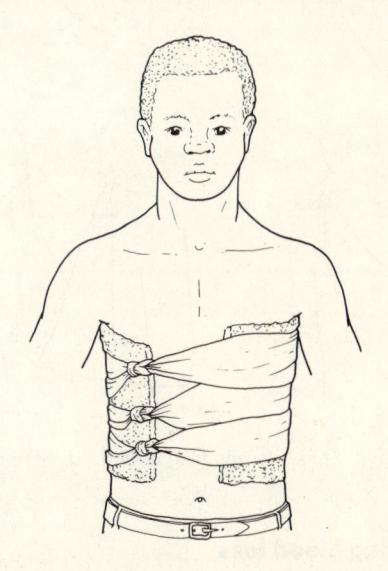

*Fig. 3.13 Using a small pillow to splint the chest*

Place the patient in the position he finds most comfortable—usually semi-recumbent (Fig. 2.18), with head and shoulders raised and the body inclined to the injured side. Support him in this position by placing rolled-up coats, blankets or pillows behind his back.

Treat him for shock until the hospital is reached.

## Bleeding from the palm of the hand

Apply direct pressure.
Raise the arm.
If no fracture or foreign body, such as a piece of glass you cannot remove, is present:

- cover the wound with a clean dressing;
- place a pad over the dressing;
- bend the patient's fingers over the pad;
- bandage the fist firmly;
- support the limb in a sling (Fig. 3.14);
- refer to health centre or hospital.

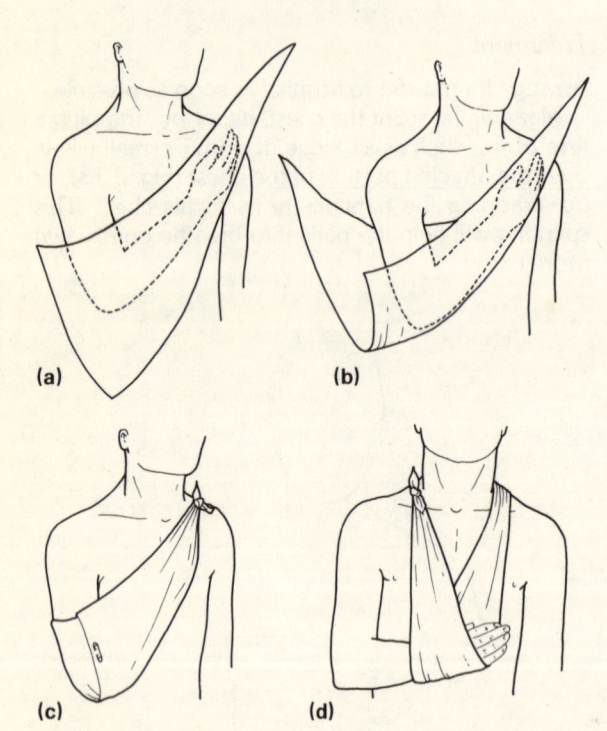

*Fig. 3.14 a–c. Stages in applying a sling. d. Simple hand sling*

## Estimating blood loss

It helps to know the amount of blood which needs to be given to a patient, if you can give some idea of the amount of blood lost at the scene of an accident and report this to the hospital or health centre.

For bleeding from the ear, nose, tooth socket, tongue, and cheek, see pages 83–84.

## Bandages and bandaging

A bandage has two main purposes: first to keep a splint or dressing in place, and second to apply pressure.

If the bandage you have is dirty or wet, it is better to apply no bandage at all.

Cloth kept for bandaging should be washed and dried with an iron or placed in the sun in a clean, dust-free place.

If possible, always cover the wound with a sterile gauze pad before bandaging. These pads are sold in sealed envelopes in the majority of pharmacies. You can also make your own gauze or cloth sterile. Wrap it in thick paper, seal it with tape and bake it in an oven for 20 minutes (a pan of water in the oven under the cloth will prevent it from burning or smouldering).

### Bandages to keep a dressing in place

Any clean material which will go right round the wounded part and keep the dressing in place can be used—a scarf, stocking or tie, as well as the more usual bandages which can be bought in pharmacies.

### Bandages to apply pressure

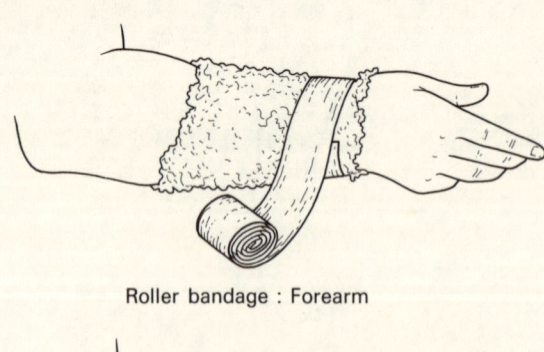

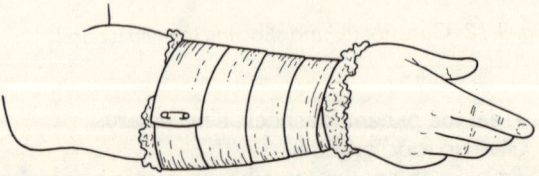

*Fig. 3.15 Bandaging to apply pressure*

Firm, even pressure is best applied by a crêpe bandage that is fairly well stretched as it is being put on. You can get even pressure by applying the bandage over a thick layer of wool extending well over the wound (Fig. 3.15).

If elastic bandages containing rubber are used, they require special care; they should be stretched only slightly when being put on. If possible they should be avoided altogether.

*Pressure dressings for large wounds*

These can be made of layers of gauze (or clean linen) and cotton wool bandaged in position (Fig. 3.16).

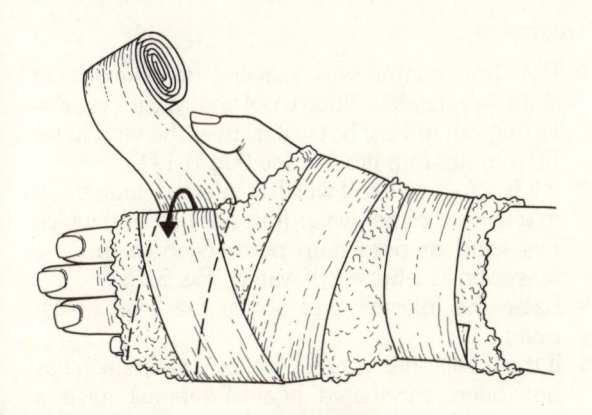

Roller bandage: Hand

*Fig. 3.16 Pressure dressing for a large wound*

*Emergency dressings*

These can be made from clean linen or a towel, or a handkerchief which (preferably) has been well ironed (the heat will kill many germs).

Hold up the material by its corners and allow it to fall open: then refold it without touching the surface which previously was inside but is now outside.

Place the dressing over the wound.

Secure in place by using any suitable strip of cloth available (e.g. tie, scarf, etc.).

## Local cures for treating wounds

Some infusions made from the barks of local trees are used for treating wounds. Be absolutely sure they are safe, clean, and do good before using them.

Never use animal or human faeces or dirt—these can cause dangerous infections, including tetanus.

Alcohol, tincture of iodine, etc. applied directly on an open wound will damage the flesh and delay healing.

Never use dirty water on open wounds. It is better not to wash them at all if that is all you can get.

If no clean boiled water is available for washing wounds, the juice of some cactus plants can be used.

## Wounds which are likely to become infected

- Dirty wounds.
- Wounds made with dirty objects, e.g. a used knife or needle for ear or nose piercing.
- Puncture wounds.
- Deep wounds which do not bleed much.
- Wounds which occur where animals are kept: pig pens, corrals, etc.
- Large wounds with severe bruising or crushing.
- Bites from people and animals.
- Bullet wounds.
- Baby's cord if cut with dirty scissors or knife (seek medical advice quickly for this infection).

## Special care for dirty wounds

- Wash the wound well with boiled clean water and soap. Remove all bits of dirt, blood clots, dead or badly damaged flesh. Flood out the wound with boiled water.
- Soak the wound in water to which potassium permanganate has been added (1 teaspoonful potassium permanganate to 1 bucket of water).
- Paint the wound with gentian violet or put antibiotic ointment on the wound.
- Cover with a clean bandage.
- If the wound is very deep, is a bite, or if there is the slightest chance that it still has dirt in it, give an antibiotic (for dosages see the pharmacopoeia).
- **Never** close this type of wound with stitches or butterfly sutures. **Leave the wound open**.
- Contact your supervisor for advice.

## Tetanus risk

Tetanus is caused by a germ which lives in the stools of animals or people and enters the body through a wound.

The danger of tetanus is very great to a person who has not been vaccinated against it. Give him penicillin or ampicillin even if his wound is small.

If the wound is large and severe, a person who has not been vaccinated against tetanus should take large doses of penicillin or ampicillin for at least a week.

If tetanus antitoxin is given, all necessary precautions must be taken. Contact your supervisor for advice.

## Some of the dangers of injecting certain medicines such as antibiotics and antitoxins

The following groups of medicines sometimes produce a dangerous reaction called allergic shock a short time after being injected into the patient:

- penicillins (including ampicillin);
- antitoxins that are made from horse serum: scorpion antivenom; snake antivenom; tetanus antitoxin.

The risk of a serious reaction is greater in a person who has already been injected with one of these medicines or with another in the same group. The risk is especially great if the previous injection caused irritation, a rash, swelling or difficulty in breathing within a few hours or some days later.

To prevent a serious reaction from an injection:

- Use injections only when absolutely necessary.
- Before injecting one of the medicines listed above, have ready 2 ampoules of adrenaline and 1 ampoule of an antihistamine (phenergan or benadryl: see pharmacopoeia for dosage).
- Before giving the injection, ask whether at any time a similar injection caused illness, a rash, irritation etc. If the patient says 'yes', do **not** give this medicine **nor any other in the same group**, either by injection or by mouth.
- In very serious cases such as tetanus or snakebite, when you must give an injection, but the patient indicates that the antitoxin is likely to produce an allergic reaction, give an injection of phergan or benadryl 15 minutes before giving the antitoxin (see pharmacopoeia for dosage).
- After giving any medicine by injection, stay with the patient for at least 30 minutes. Watch for any of the following signs and symptoms or allergic shock: cold, moist, pale skin; sweating; weak rapid pulse; difficulty in breathing; loss of consciousness.
- If any of these signs and symptoms appear, immediately inject adrenaline (adult ½ ml; children ¼ ml).
- Treat the patient for shock (page 6).
- Give one of the antihistamines in double the normal dose.
- Report to your supervisor for further advice.

## Infected wounds: How to recognise them and how to treat them

A wound is infected if:

- it becomes red, swollen, hot and painful; or
- it has pus; or
- it begins to swell.

The infection is spreading to other parts of the body, if:

- it causes fever;
- there is a red line near the wound;
- the lymph glands (small nodules in the armpit; groin or neck) become swollen and painful.

*Treatment*

- Put hot compresses (several thicknesses of cloth—preferably cotton wool and gauze 'packs'—wrung out in very hot water) over the wound for 20 minutes four times a day (Fig. 3.17).
- If it is a foot or hand which is infected, immerse it in a bucket of hot water (but not **too** hot) which has soap or potassium permanganate in it—1 teaspoon to 1 bucket of water) (Fig. 3.18).
- Raise the infected part above the level of the heart.
- If the infection is very severe, or if the person has not been vaccinated against tetanus, give a course of an antibiotic such as penicillin (see pharmacopoeia).
- Seek advice from your supervisor.

### Gas gangrene

Gas gangrene is a very dangerous infection of a wound from which a foul-smelling grey or brown liquid oozes (Fig. 3.19).

The skin near the wound may have dark blisters and the flesh may have air bubbles in it.

This infection begins to appear between 6 hours and 3 days after the injury. It gets worse quickly and spreads. Without treatment it will cause death within a few days.

Get medical help or advice. If this is not possible:

- keep the patient away from others;
- open the wound;
- wash it out with boiled water and soap;
- clean out all dead and damaged flesh;
- if possible, flood the wound with hydrogen peroxide every 2 hours;
- inject penicillin (crystalline if available) one million units every 3 hours;

A Bad Cut or Wound 25

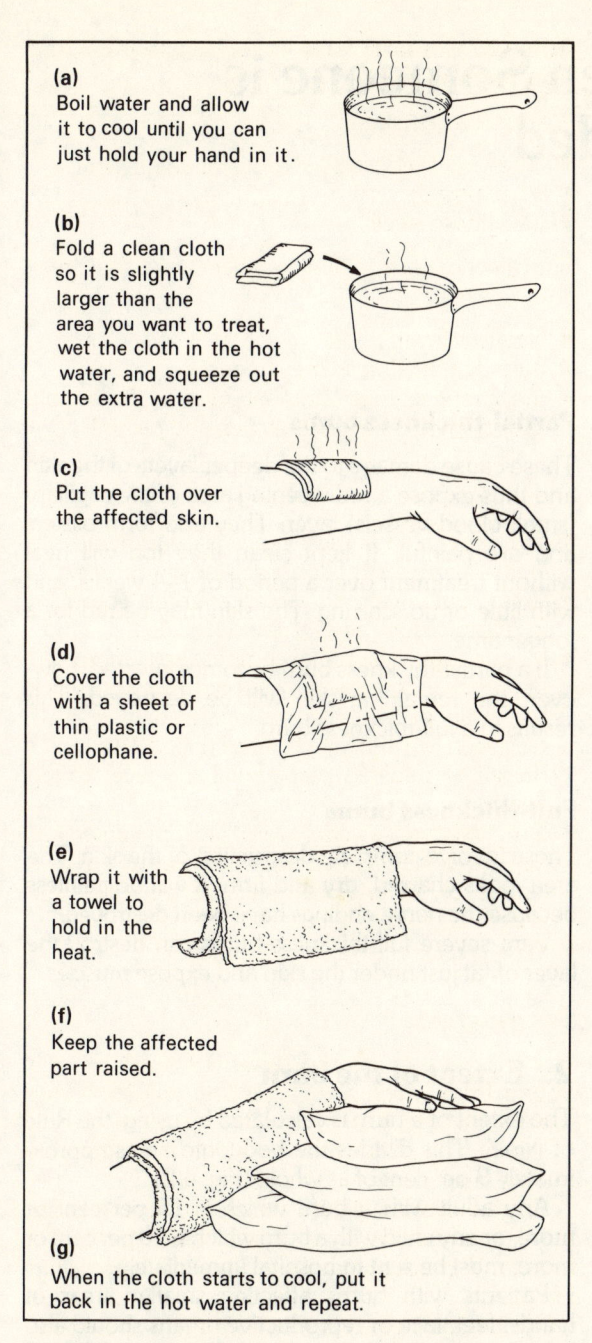

**(a)** Boil water and allow it to cool until you can just hold your hand in it.

**(b)** Fold a clean cloth so it is slightly larger than the area you want to treat, wet the cloth in the hot water, and squeeze out the extra water.

**(c)** Put the cloth over the affected skin.

**(d)** Cover the cloth with a sheet of thin plastic or cellophane.

**(e)** Wrap it with a towel to hold in the heat.

**(f)** Keep the affected part raised.

**(g)** When the cloth starts to cool, put it back in the hot water and repeat.

*Fig. 3.17 Instructions for using hot compresses*

- leave the wound uncovered so that air can get to it;
- boil all dressings and equipment you use;
- thoroughly scrub your own hands and arms with soap and water (if possible under running water);
- get medical help as soon as you can.

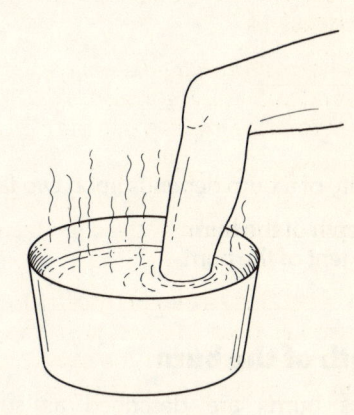

*Fig. 3.18 Hot soaks*

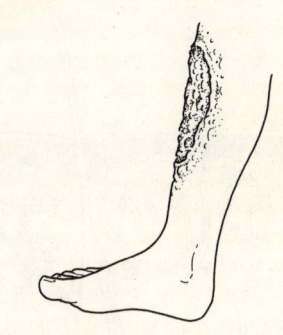

*Fig. 3.19 Gas gangrene*

# 4. What to Do when Someone is Burned or Scalded

The severity of a burn depends upon two factors:
(1) the depth of the burn;
(2) the extent of the burn.

## 1. Depth of the burn

Sometimes burns are described as superficial, partial-thickness or full-thickness (or first-degree, second-degree and third-degree) (Fig. 4.1).

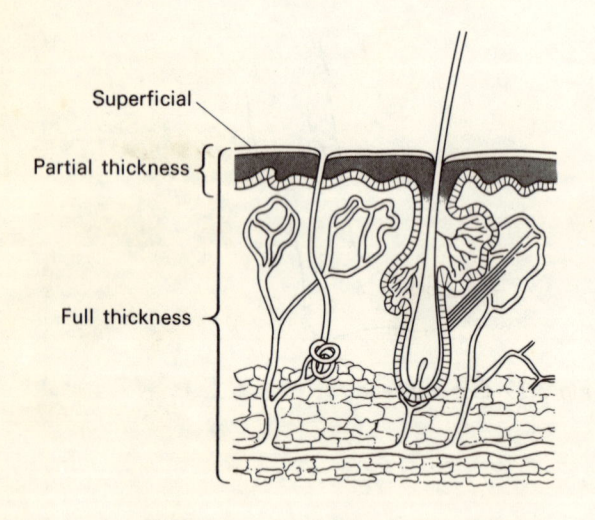

*Fig. 4.1 The skin showing various depths of burns*

### Superficial or surface burns

These are burns of the outer layer of the skin and cause blisters and reddening. They are painful because the nerve endings are irritated. They usually heal without treatment within 3 days.

### Partial-thickness burns

These cause damage to the deeper layers of the skin and thus expose a red weeping area of the capillary (small blood vessels) layer. They also form blisters and are painful. If kept clean they too will heal without treatment over a period of 1–4 weeks, and with little or no scarring. The skin may be red for a longer time.

If a partial-thickness burn becomes infected, however, the remaining skin will be destroyed. This results in a full-thickness burn.

### Full-thickness burns

These involve complete destruction of the skin. The area looks charred, dry and firm. It will be painless because the nerve endings have been destroyed.

Very severe full-thickness burns can destroy the layer of fat just under the skin and expose muscles.

## 2. Extent of the burn

The extent of a burn is calculated by using 'the Rule of Nine'. This divides the body into areas approximately 9 per cent of its whole (Fig. 4.2).

Any adult with a burn which is 15 per cent or more, or any child with a burn which is 10 per cent or more, must be sent to hospital immediately.

Patients with burns affecting smaller areas of hands, feet, face or reproductive organs should also be transported to hospital or to a health centre as soon as possible.

### Treatment of burns

If the person's clothes are on fire:
- put out the flames with cold water or sand if either is to hand;

## Burns and Scalds

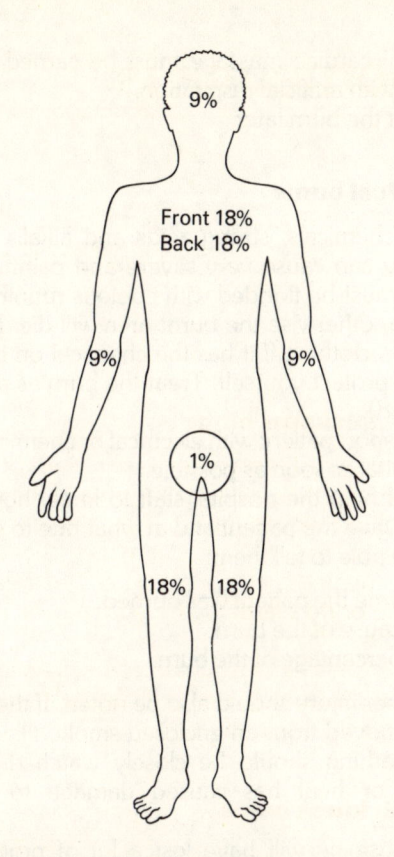

*Fig. 4.2 The 'Rule of Nine' showing how the body can be divided to calculate the area of skin burnt*

### Severe burns

The loss of fluid from the circulation into the tissues may lead to shock and swelling of the flesh.

*Treatment*

- Treat for shock.
- Wrap patient in a clean sheet and transport him to hospital as soon as possible.

Meanwhile:

- give fluids: to one litre of water add:
  ½ teaspoonful salt;
  ½ teaspoonful sodium bicarbonate;
  2–3 tablespoonfuls sugar or honey, orange or lemon juice.

Encourage the patient to drink this mixture (Fig. 4.3).

---

Give the burned person plenty of liquid. If the burned area is large (more than twice the size of his hand), make up the following drink:

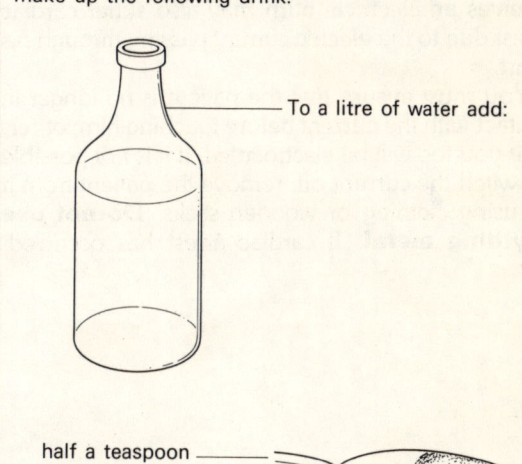

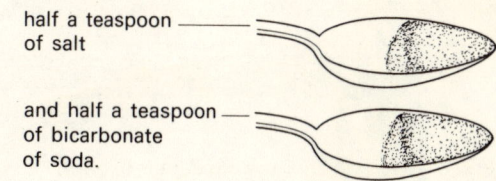

To a litre of water add:

half a teaspoon of salt

and half a teaspoon of bicarbonate of soda.

Also put in 2 or 3 tablespoons of sugar or honey and some orange or lemon juice if possible.

The burned person should drink this as often as possible, especially until he urinates frequently.

---

- if water is not available, smother the flames by laying the victim down and wrapping a blanket, coat or rug very lightly around him;
- tear off smouldering clothing by seizing the non-burning areas of material;
- immerse or flood the affected part in cold water;
- remove any clothing which is soaked in boiling water, oil or other fluid;
- do **not** remove burnt clothing which has cooled;
- remove any constricting items such as shoes, boots, rings and bracelets before swelling begins;
- cover the area **lightly** with a sterile or very clean cloth or sheet.

**Do not**:

- handle the burned areas;
- prick any blisters;
- apply lotion or ointment;
- remove skin or pieces of cloth etc. which are stuck to the burnt skin.

*Fig. 4.3 Making up a mixture for a badly burned patient to drink*

- Comfort and give him confidence that you know what you are doing;
- Give aspirin or codeine to relieve pain.

## Minor burns and scalds

*Treatment*

- Place the affected part under clean running water if possible. If a tap is not available, get a bucket of very cold water and plunge the burned or scalded part of the body into this.
- Repeat every 3–4 minutes until the burn is no longer painful when out of water.
- It is important to keep all burns **very clean** to prevent infection.

## Electrical burns

Electrical burns are usually deep. A patient who receives an electrical burn may also suffer cardiac arrest due to the electric current passing through his heart.

You must ensure that the patient is no longer in contact with the current before touching him; otherwise you too will be electrocuted. If it is not possible to switch the current off; remove the patient from it by using clothing or wooden sticks. **Do not use anything metal**. If cardiac arrest has occurred, external cardiac massage must be carried out, together with artificial respiration.

Treat the burn later.

## Chemical burns

Some chemicals, strong acids and alkalis used in industry can cause very severe and painful burns. These must be flooded with copious running water at once, otherwise the burnt area will die. Remove patient's clothing if it has the chemical on it, taking care to protect yourself. Treat the burn as a wound (page 18).

Transport patient with electrical or chemical burns to hospital as soon as possible.

It will help the hospital staff to know how much fluid to give the patient and at what rate to give it, if you are able to tell them:

- the time the patient was burned;
- the cause of the burn;
- the percentage of the burn.

Any other injury should also be noted. If the patient was removed from an enclosed smoke-filled room, his breathing should be closely watched in case smoke or heat has caused damage to the air passages.

Because he will have lost a lot of protein, the burned patient during his convalescence should be encouraged to eat a lot of meat, fish, soya beans, cheese, etc.

# 5. What to Do when Someone Cannot be Woken Up

There are many causes of loss of consciousness. Some of the more common ones include hysteria, belief in witchcraft, fear, etc., excessive drinking of alcohol, diabetes mellitus (sugar diabetes), fainting, a stroke or a knock on the head (causing concussion).

*Treatment*

In every case the aims are:
- to ensure that the patient can breathe (i.e. that there is a clear airway) (page 10);
- to give artificial respiration and cardiac massage if breathing and the heart stop (page 10);
- to prevent further injury; and
- to obtain medical help as soon as possible.

## Loss of consciousness due to fainting

Fainting occurs when the brain does not receive enough blood for its needs. This may happen to someone who has had severe diarrhoea and vomiting; who has seen or heard something upsetting; or who has stood for a long time in hot and crowded circumstances. The victim will be pale, sweaty and will fall to the ground as he loses consciousness.

*Treatment*

Once he is in a horizontal position the patient is likely to recover fairly quickly, because the blood supply to his brain will improve. He should be kept flat, therefore, and should not attempt to sit up until he is fully recovered. If the faint occurs in a crowd it may be a good idea to transfer him outside to fresh air. When conscious, he may be given a drink of water.

## Loss of consciousness attributed to witchcraft or black magic or the evil eye (hysteria)

If someone believes strongly enough that a witch has power to harm, he may become ill or go into a deep sleep. But anyone in this state is the victim of his own fear. A 'witch' has no power over people, except for the ability to make them believe that she has. For this reason it is impossible to bewitch a person who does not believe in witchcraft.

As a community health worker it is one of your responsibilities to help people to understand the real causes of illness and disease, and that such sicknesses have nothing to do with witchcraft or black magic.

While many home remedies or traditional cures have a good and direct effect on the body, others work only because people believe in them—just as bewitching works when people believe in that. For this reason, someone who believes in witchcraft is likely to have sufficient faith in the home cure to make it work. Find out what is believed locally to help to awaken people, and use it. Remember even when people appear to be sound asleep often they can still hear, so speak of the home cure into the person's ear. In this kind of treatment it is the manner or touch of the first-aider which can be important: show that you care; say that you believe he will recover quickly; give him confidence that all will soon be well, and that he has nothing to be afraid of.

## Loss of consciousness due to drunkenness

Too much alcohol is a well-known cause of deep sleep. A little alcohol now and again does no harm, but a lot of alcohol does a lot of harm and in time leads to death. Heavy drinking of alcohol is one of the main causes of many health problems, not only of the person who drinks but also of his family and the community. As a community health worker it is one of your responsibilities to help people to understand that too much alcohol can harm the health and happiness of everyone around.

If drink is the cause of the deep sleep, you will be able to smell it on the breath of, and around, the sleeper. He will need to 'sleep it off'. When conscious, black coffee may help him to come back to normal more quickly. After that he will need your help in deciding to cut down on the amount he drinks. A few people are able simply to decide that they will stop drinking altogether. More often people need help from their family, friends and others who can understand how hard it is to give up the habit. People who have been heavy drinkers and have stopped are often the best persons to help others to do the same.

## Loss of consciousness due to diabetes mellitus (sugar diabetes)

The onset of diabetes mellitus is a gradual process. The person feels very thirsty, drinks more than before, passes more urine than before, loses weight and feels unwell. If all these symptoms are ignored, in time he can lapse into coma (deep unconsciousness). He will be in urgent need of medical assistance and this should be obtained as soon as possible. Again, it is a time for contacting your supervisor for advice and then transporting the patient to a hospital.

*Treatment*

Because in diabetes the patient's body is not producing enough of a substance called insulin, in order to digest all the food he eats, the treatment is to give him insulin, usually by injection (sometimes in tablet form). Once a balance of food and insulin has been worked out, the person is able to live a normal life with the diabetes under control but not cured. If something upsets this balance between food and insulin, a state of deep unconsciousness (coma) may develop.

A difficulty is to decide whether the diabetic person who is in coma has had too much insulin for the food to use, or whether he has had too much food for the insulin to cope with. If someone whom you know to be a diabetic feels faint, begins to sweat, looks ill and becomes mentally confused, give him sugar at once. This can be ordinary sugar, glucose, a spoonful of honey or a sweet drink.

If the coma is due to too much insulin the person will begin to recover at once. If it is due to too much sugar the small amount you have given will do no harm but you must get medical assistance at once.

The main difference between the two kinds of coma are shown in Table 5.1.

**TABLE 5.1. Differences between Insulin and Diabetic comas**

|  | INSULIN COMA | DIABETIC COMA |
|---|---|---|
| History: | No food intake, but Insulin taken. | Food. Insulin or no Insulin taken. |
| Onset: | Immediately before the onset in good health. The onset is related to time of last injection of Insulin. | In poor health for several days. |
| Signs: | Moist skin and tongue. Normal or raised blood pressure. Shallow or normal breathing. Full pulse. Improves immediately after given some sugar or sweets. | Dry skin and tongue. Low blood pressure. Laboured breathing (Air hunger—apple odour). Weak pulse. |

## Loss of consciousness due to a stroke

All our body movements and functions (workings) are controlled by the brain, which is a very complex organ. Like all organs it requires a good supply of blood in order to work: the supply has to be sufficient and steady. Any alteration in this supply will show itself by a loss of function (working) or loss of movement of some part of the body. Sometimes bleeding, or a clot of blood, causes a brain illness, known as a stroke.

Strokes vary according to the size of the area of the brain which is affected. They range from very short periods of loss of consciousness, followed by numbness or tingling of a few muscles, to such severe damage that the patient never regains consciousness and dies.

In the majority of instances the patient loses consciousness for a time and then regains it. Often he is left with a degree of paralysis of one side of the body and sometimes his speech is slurred.

*Treatment*

- First aid is the same as that for anyone who has become unconscious.
- First, it is essential to check that the patient is breathing. If not, artificial respiration must be started (see page 10), and if necessary and appropriate (i.e. within 3 minutes of the cessation of the heart beating), heart massage also (see page 14).
- Send for help and advice.
- Stay with the patient and place him in as comfortable a position as possible.
- Keep him quiet and still until medical assistance arrives.

## Loss of consciousness due to a heart attack

Unconsciousness sometimes occurs during a heart attack (for treatment see page 14).

## Loss of consciousness due to a knock on the head (causing concussion)

After a knock on the head there may be some loss of consciousness and also some loss of memory. The latter may be for a brief time only. The cause is usually a direct blow to the jaw or skull. This can happen in a fall or during some sport, e.g. football or in a fight.

*Signs and symptoms*

- Mild mental confusion.
- Some brief loss of memory.
- Difficulty with seeing.
- Headache.
- Nausea (feeling sick).
- Irritability (sometimes).
- A change in the level of consciousness (see page 4).

*Treatment*

- Keep the patient resting and quiet.
- Do not leave him alone.
- Do **not** give alcohol, medicine to relieve pain or sleeping pills.
- Transport to hospital as soon as possible or contact your supervisor for advice.

## Loss of consciousness due to poisoning

This is dealt with in detail in the next chapter (see pages 32–39).

# 6. What to Do when Someone Swallows Poison or is Poisoned by a Sting or Bite

The treatment of a poisoned person is a matter of extreme urgency.
**You must act at once: get the poisoned person to hospital or health centre immediately.**
The most common types of poisoning occur when poisonous substances are swallowed (or enter the digestive system). Food poisoning is probably the most common of all. All types of poisoning—whether it is kerosene being swallowed by a child who thinks it is water, or an overdose of a medicine—can threaten life. The extent of the danger depends upon:

- the amount and type of poison, drug or medicine taken;
- the age of the person;
- whether the person vomits;
- where the accident takes place.

## General signs and symptoms of sudden poisoning

- Nausea.
- Vomiting.
- Belly pains.
- Change in degree of consciousness (see page 4).
- Changes in breathing (either an increase or decrease in depth and rate).
- Changes in pulse (either an increase or decrease in rate and strength).
- Changes in pupils (either larger or smaller).
- Convulsions (fits).

## Most usual ways of poisoning

- By ingestion (through the mouth), e.g. infected food or water.
- By inhalation (by being breathed in), e.g. fumes from motor-car or gas.
- By absorption (through the skin), e.g. snake bites or insect stings.

Because different poisons result in different signs and symptoms, it is difficult to give precise ones for every poison. Again 'clues' can be useful in helping you to know which one you are dealing with. So in any suspected case of poisoning:

- look for physical changes as described above;
- look for burns or stains on the face, particularly around the mouth;
- smell the breath;
- make a quick check of the surroundings for empty pill boxes, bottles, sprays, plants, berries, etc.

If you can quickly discover the source of the poison, take it with the patient to hospital or medical help. It will help the staff to know which antidote (the 'opposite' substance which will neutralise the poison) to give.

The steps of treatment are:

- to remove the poison from the body;
- to give the patient the antidote (a substance which will neutralise the poison) for the poison—if you know it; if not, give a soothing mixture (see below);
- to treat symptoms;
- to give comfort and confidence throughout.

In hospital, the poison is usually removed from the stomach (belly) by washing it out, but this is not done if the poison is one which burns (e.g. a corrosive) or one which induces fits (e.g. strychnine).

If you have to treat the poisoned person yourself, in most cases you can try to remove the poison from his body by making him vomit it. Give him a drink of tepid water with mustard or soap in it. Children can be made to vomit by giving them syrup of ipecac 15 ml. Repeat the procedure of making the patient vomit until the vomit is clear.

**Do not** make the patient vomit if the poison is one which burns, or if it is petrol or kerosene. Instead, give milk with egg whites or a mixture of flour and water.

**Do not** make the patient vomit if he is unconscious.

Cover him if he feels cold, but avoid too much heat.

## Antidotes (substances which neutralise the poison)

If you know the poison is an acid, give the opposite—an alkali—e.g. sodium bicarbonate. If the poison is an alkali give the opposite—an acid—e.g. vinegar.

The following are a few antidotes which may be found in the household:

- for poisoning by a metal, e.g. iron, give milk and egg whites;
- for poisoning by an irritant, e.g. iodine, give flour or starch water;
- for poisoning by an alkaloid give strong tea, or diluted tincture of iodine.

Substances which are meant to poison usually have the antidote printed on the label. Again it is emphasised, unless you are far from a hospital, do not waste time in hunting for an antidote—take the patient to medical help.

Many swallowed poisons are excreted by the kidneys, so it is good practice to give lots of fluids and to encourage the person to continue to drink a lot of water for at least 24 hours after being poisoned.

## Specific poisons and their effects

### Acids

Battery acid is very poisonous. It is colourless and if kept in an unlabelled bottle can easily be mistaken for glycerine. When swallowed it burns the mouth and tongue and causes great pain. The victim will collapse and need treating for shock. This should be given on the way to medical aid.

### Alkalis

Caustic soda may be mistaken for a laxative. It causes swelling of the lips and tongue and burning pain from mouth to belly. The victim will retch and vomit. Shock is usually severe and the patient will need to be treated for that at once.

Ammonia is often stored in the home or workplace. If fumes from ammonia get into the eyes, they can cause severe irritation, pain and permanent damage. The eyes must be flushed out at once—the quickest way is to plunge the patient's whole face into a bowl of tepid water and tell him to open and close his eyes.

### Antihistamines (medicines given for an allergy (sensitivity))

Children sometimes mistake these brightly coloured pills for sweets. They should be kept in a cupboard which is locked, or at least out of their reach.

The most common effects of these medicines are drowsiness or sleep. There may also be giddiness, headache, dry mouth and sometimes vomiting and diarrhoea.

If a large amount has been swallowed, breathing may stop and mouth-to-mouth respiration will be needed.

### Aspirin

The fatal dose of aspirin varies considerably. Moderate overdoses cause nausea (a feeling of sickness) and tinnitus (ringing in the ears). Deafness may occur later. Larger doses cause mental confusion, drowsiness or unconsciousness (coma). The patient will sweat profusely and may vomit blood.

### Sleeping pills (sedatives)

While there are very many sleeping pills, they can be divided very roughly into those which act quickly and last a short time and those which act slowly and last for a longer time. Some sedatives contain ingredients which do both. When too large a dose has been taken, the first effects are giddiness, headache, and being unable to stand or walk without falling.

Before sleep comes, the patient may be excitable and talk a lot. His breathing may be noisy. The pupils of his eyes will be small but not as small as pin-points (morphine or heroin poisoning).

### Insecticides

Many insecticides when swallowed will cause aching in the limbs, weakness of the muscles and sometimes fits (see page 62).

Poisoning by strychnine causes very intense pain and spasms (tightenings) of the muscles.

## Iron

Again, because iron tablets are an attractive colour, children often think they are sweets. If a large quantity is eaten it can be very dangerous. The child will become pale and vomit (sometimes blood). If he is not made to vomit them all, he will become shocked, very drowsy and restless.

## Lead

Chronic (long-term and coming on gradually) lead poisoning can happen to children who bite or suck railings, cot bars or paint, etc. which contains lead. They become irritable, drowsy and constipated. They may also have headaches and colicky pain (sharp pain for short periods which comes and goes).

## Lysol

This is a corrosive poison which burns the tongue and mouth. Although there is pain to begin with, this disappears after a time as it has an anaesthetic (numbing) effect.

The patient collapses and becomes unconscious. As he is likely to vomit, it is important to treat him in the recovery position (Fig. 2.6).

## Mercury

Some seed dressings and insecticides used on the land contain mercury. The first symptoms of poisoning will be irritation and a feeling of heat in the throat. The patient may also vomit and sometimes faint. Later severe abdominal (belly) pain will occur and much later, diarrhoea (passing of loose, watery stools).

## Paraffin and petrol (gasoline)

Paraffin and petrol are sometimes swallowed accidentally by children. The immediate effects are restlessness, vomiting and diarrhoea. The child may become drowsy or have fits, or both.

## Weedkillers

Arsenic is often present in weedkillers, some sprays used for agricultural purposes, the powders used for destroying ant-hills, and also in other similar preparations which are used in the house. Store and use all these with great care.

Arsenic is tasteless. Symptoms of poisoning are similar to those of mercury poisoning.

It is important to be able to tell the difference between food poisoning and metal poisoning. Whereas in food poisoning vomiting stops fairly soon, in mercury and arsenic poisoning it continues. In food poisoning diarrhoea begins early, but in mercury and arsenic poisoning it may not happen for as long as 12 hours.

Sodium chlorate is the least harmful weedkiller for general use. Those containing paraquat are safe if the instructions which are given are carefully followed. If accidentally swallowed, paraquat causes headaches, tight chest pains and a strong dislike of light (photophobia).

## Poisoning through the skin

If the poison has not been swallowed, but has been in contact with the skin, repeated bathing in running water is the most effective treatment.

If the irritant does not dissolve in water, use vegetable oil or alcohol instead.

When you suspect that an area of skin has been in contact with a poisonous plant, scrub the skin with soap and water.

## Poisons which are inhaled (breathed in)

### Gas poisoning

Remove the patient into fresh air to help get rid of the gas in his lungs and also to lessen the risk of injury from explosions.

Mouth-to-mouth respiration and cardiac massage must be given immediately if necessary (see page 14).

It is vital for you to draw well clear of the patient between breaths so that your breathed-in air does not become contaminated by his breath.

Recovery from the effects of gas poisoning is fairly slow and you have to continue mouth-to-mouth breathing for some time.

**Never** use a flame anywhere near gas.

## Poisoning by plants

Each country has some trees and plants, some parts of which are poisonous; e.g. bark, berries, fruits, leaves, juice, roots or stalk.

It is important to know which these are, to teach people (especially children) which they are, and to know how to treat people who swallow the poisonous part by accident. Many good traditional cures will be known locally.

## Poisoning by snakes

A snake bite can be dangerous and may cause death. Again, in many villages, people often know how to treat snake bites and it is well worthwhile getting to know them yourself (Fig. 6.1). If you have no anti-venom (the antidote), traditional methods—such as porous stone applied to the bite—may work well.

**(a) Poisonous snake**

Fang marks.

The bite of a poisonous snake leaves marks of the 2 fangs (and at rare times, other little marks made by the teeth).

**(b) Non-poisonous snake**

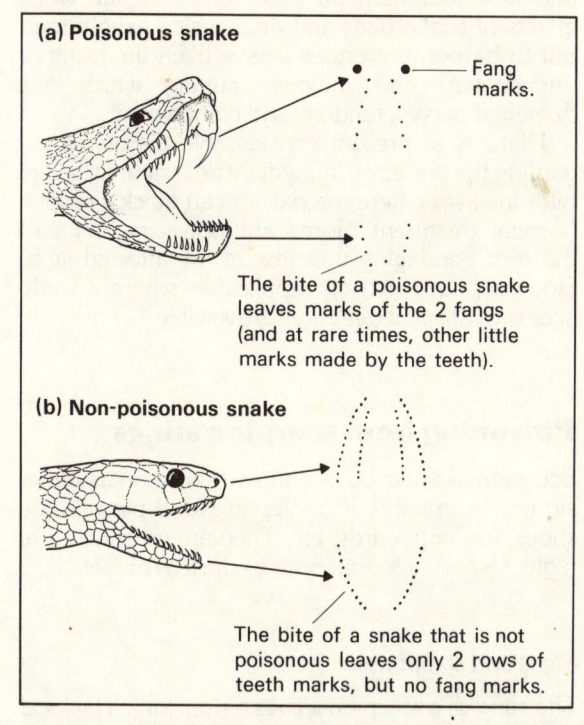

The bite of a snake that is not poisonous leaves only 2 rows of teeth marks, but no fang marks.

*Fig. 6.1 (a) Poisonous and (b) nonpoisonous snake bites*

Most snake bites occur in daylight and on the foot or ankle because the victim treads on or near the snake. The effect of the bite depends mainly upon the amount of venom injected. Snakes frequently bite without injecting venom.

Fright, especially the fear of a rapid and unpleasant death, is the most common symptom following a snake bite. It is important to distinguish symptoms of fear—faintness, stupor, cold, clammy skin, feeble pulse and rapid shallow breathing—from those of poisoning by venom. Emotional symptoms come on immediately. Symptoms from poisoning rarely begin until ½ to 1 hour after the bite.

Local swelling with pain follows viper bites if venom has been injected. If there is no swelling and the snake which bit is known to be a viper, poisoning has not taken place. The amount of swelling in a viper bite depends upon the amount of venom injected. If swelling extends above the knee (or above the elbow if a hand has been bitten) there is considerable poisoning. Blisters forming on a limb are a sign that a high dose of venom has been injected into the patient.

Swelling from cobra venom develops more slowly, taking 1–2 hours.

In sea-snake poisoning, the patient's muscles become paralysed. Limb, neck and body movements may all become very painful. This will be followed by shock and collapse. Mouth-to-mouth respiration and heart massage may be given, but the outlook is serious.

The fangs of certain cobras in Africa are so designed that venom can be spat out at right angles. The stream of venom may squirt up to a height of 6 feet and may strike the victim's face and eyes. This causes very painful inflammation. The eyes should be washed out immediately with clean water or boric acid solution (1 teaspoonful to 1 pint of warm water).

### General treatment of snake bites

Calm the victim.

Apply a firm, but not tight cord just above the bite. **This must be removed within 15 minutes**, or when you have reached medical assistance, whichever is the shortest time.

Wipe the wound of venom which may have spilled from the fangs at the time of biting.

Get the patient to hospital immediately, or as soon as possible. If it is considered necessary, appropriate anti-venom will be given with proper precautions.

### Specific treatment of a snake bite with poisoning

If you are sure that venom has been injected and you cannot get the victim to hospital in time, **only then** should you carry out the following treatment:

- tie a cord tightly around the limb just above the bite (Fig. 6.2(a));
- using a razor blade or a clean knife, make a cut 1 cm deep (Fig. 6.2(b));

## 36  First Aid

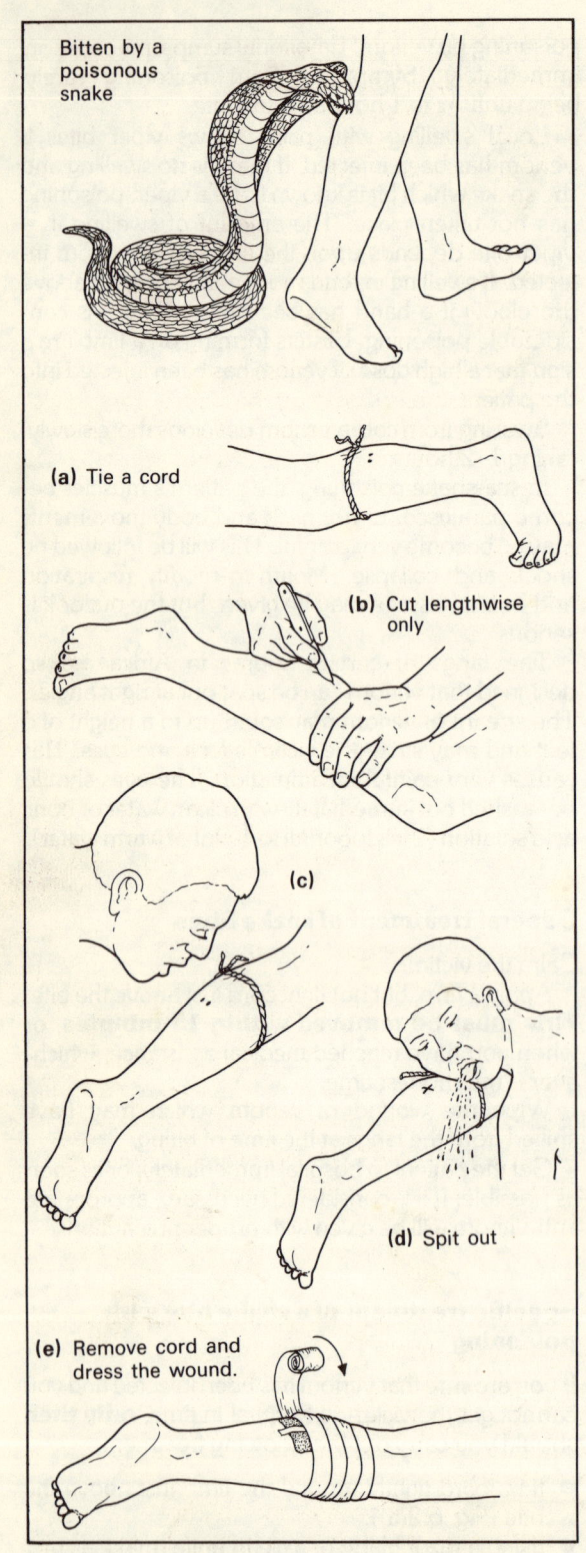

**Fig. 6.2** Treating a bite from a poisonous snake

(a) Tie a cord
(b) Cut lengthwise only
(c)
(d) Spit out
(e) Remove cord and dress the wound.

- suck the liquid which is coming out of the wound (Fig. 6.2(c));
- spit out the liquid immediately (Fig. 6.2(d));
- continue to suck and spit for 5–10 minutes;
- loosen the cord tie around the patient's limb;
- disinfect the wound;
- bandage the wound (Fig. 6.2(e));
- give an anti-venom injection if you have it.

Proper precautions must be taken in case the patient is sensitive to the serum. Test this by giving 0.1 ml just under the skin. If there is sensitivity (allergic reaction) give the anti-venom in gradually increasing doses. Only in extreme life-and-death cases should the full injection, without testing, be given.

Likewise only in extreme cases should the cut-and-suck treatment be used. Some of the worst effects of snake bites and ones which have turned out to be non-poisonous—have been the result of unnecessary and inexpert cutting which has damaged nerves, tendons and blood vessels.

There is at present considerable discussion regarding the preferred immediate treatment for snake bites in cases where the patient can quickly receive hospital treatment. Some authorities recommend the firm bandaging upwards of the affected limb. However, this is only applicable where speedy access to hospital treatment is available.

## Poisoning from scorpion stings

Scorpions shelter by day in warm dry areas under stones, in crevices in rocks, in wood-piles, inside shoes and cupboards, etc. They are most active at night. Usually a scorpion stings the legs or feet.

*Signs and symptoms*

The sting of a scorpion leaves a puncture. The local reaction is immediate and may be extremely painful. A red mark appears at the site; the area around it becomes very swollen and there may be some oozing of blood.

- The patient's pulse rate will be slow.
- His eyes and nose produce a lot of water.
- He may sneeze many times.
- He will probably sweat a lot and become very pale.
- He may feel or be sick.
- The pupils of his eyes will become dilated (large) (page 4).

*Poison, Poisonous Bites, and Stings* 37

- He is likely to complain bitterly of the pain, dizziness, trembling, headache and restlessness.
- He may lapse into unconsciousness (coma).

Get medical help at once.

*Treatment*

It is vital to have knowledge of the local kind of scorpion and the availability of anti-venom in the district.

- Rapid local relief may be obtained by injecting lignocaine or emetine around the site of the sting.
- Treat for shock.
- If you know how to do it, administer the specific anti-venom intravenously.
- For numbness and pain (which may last for weeks), hot compresses should be applied to the area (see page 24).
- Pain-killers such as aspirin may also be given.

## Poisoning from spider bites

Many spiders have poison fangs but few are strong enough to inject venom through the skin of a human being. The bites of some, however, can cause death. You should know the poisonous spiders in your district and also the local antidotes for their bites.

The best-known poisonous spider is the Black Widow, which is found in many parts of the world. Human beings are bitten only by the female. Its body is round and about ½ inch long, the belly large, black and shiny, with a red hour-glass pattern. Its web is coarse and irregular and contains a tube in which the spider hides. It is frequently found in outhouses such as outdoor privies.

*Signs and symptoms*

- There may be stinging pain, redness and swelling of the area.
- Severe pain around the bitten area will spread rapidly to muscles of the chest, belly and limbs.
- There will be severe muscle spasms (tightenings) causing the patient to double up.
- Fits are common and severe.
- The pupils of his eyes will become constricted (smaller) (see page 4).
- There will be excessive sweating and a lot of saliva will be produced.
- An adult patient may collapse and require treatment for shock, but death occurs usually only in very young children.

*Treatment*

- Anti-venom intravenously.
- Treatment for shock.
- Hot baths to relieve spasms.
- Aspirin to relieve pain.

## Poisoning from jelly-fish, some shell-fish and other fish

### Jelly-fish

Jelly-fish stings usually cause pain which is only superficial (surface), but it can be severe. The patient may require treatment for shock. The most common jelly-fish which sting are the Portuguese Man-O-War and sea wasps.

*Treatment*

- Remove tentacles holding a piece of material, or wearing a glove.
- Apply alcohol or 10 per cent formaldehyde to the stung area; if these are not available, dry sand may be sprinkled on the sting.
- If the patient collapses, tie a tourniquet round the limb but for no longer than 15 minutes or until help is obtained, whichever is the shorter time. (The tourniquet can be made from a strip of material or tie.) It will help to delay absorption of the venom.
- You may have to give mouth-to-mouth respiration and external heart massage.
- Sea wasp anti-venom is available in some countries. If it is, give that for sea wasp stings.

### Shell-fish

Poisoning from eating shell-fish has been reported from many areas of the world. The fish which most often poison are snappers, groupers, barracuda and eels.

*Signs and symptoms*

The effects of this poisoning come on soon after the fish has been eaten. They include:

- nausea and vomiting;
- profuse sweating;
- numbness of lips and throat;
- belly cramps;
- weakness of the muscles and collapse;
- death may occur from paralysis of the chest muscles necessary for breathing.

## Poisonous fish

There are many poisonous fish and they are usually found in-shore, on reefs, or buried in sand or mud. These include the stone and scorpion fish found on coral reefs and in shallow sandy waters. The injury is caused by the spines piercing the person's skin when he treads upon the fish. In some waters the sting ray causes poisoning by piercing flesh with the barbed spines of its thin waving tail.

*Signs and symptoms*

There is usually immediate pain, redness and swelling around the site of the puncture.

*Treatment*

- The most effective treatment is hot water. The part of the body which has been stung should be plunged into water as hot as the patient can bear (and only the patient can decide what that is). The pain will be relieved within seconds and the part stung must be removed from the water to avoid blistering.
- It should be plunged back into the hot water again as pain returns (within seconds at first, later within minutes).
- This procedure should be continued until the pain does not return (usually about ½ hour).
- It is important to explain the treatment to the patient, who should be given a can of boiling water to 'top up' the hot bath so that it is *constantly* as hot as he can bear.
- If the water is not hot enough, it will do no good. If the stung part is held too long in the hot water it will blister.
- If the part stung cannot be plunged into very hot water (e.g. the face), intramuscular pain killers such as pethidine should be given (see pharmacopoeia for use and dosage).

## Illness through a dog bite

The bite of a dog with a certain sickness (rabies) can cause an illness very much like poisoning (Fig. 6.3).

Rabies is a sickness due to an infection from an animal, usually a rabid dog, cat, fox, wolf, skunk, or jackal. Bats and other animals may also spread rabies. The infection grows in the animal's nerves and if its saliva enters a wound or scratch on a human being that person may develop the disease.

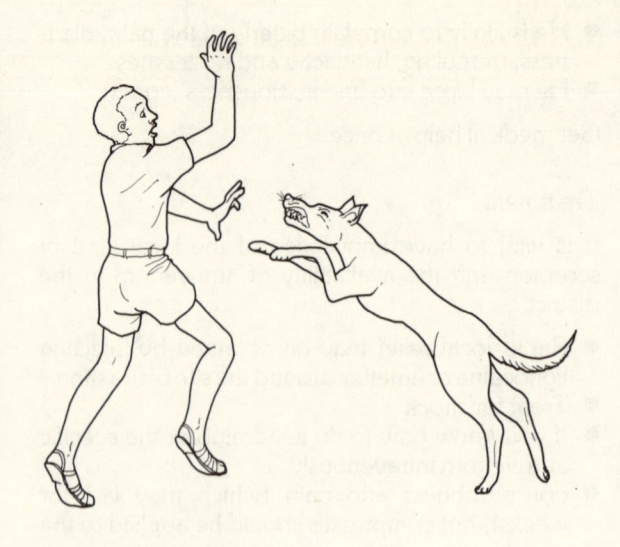

*Fig. 6.3 A Rabid dog*

If a patient has been bitten by a dog:
- clean the wound with soap and water;
- cover the wound with iodine and put on a dressing;
- bandage;
- do not close the wound;
- find out if anyone knows the dog that bit the patient;
- if someone knows it, ask: (a) if it has stopped eating ordinary food, (b) if it barks in a usual way, (c) if it trembles, is savage or never stops barking, (d) if it has fits and whether saliva runs out of its mouth;
- if the answer is 'yes' to any of these questions: (a) get the dog killed; (b) send the person to the hospital or health centre for vaccine treatment at once;
- if the dog shows none of these symptoms, ask the owner to watch the dog carefully for 10 days and to let you know if it shows any of these signs or symptoms in that time;
- if, during that time, it begins to show any of them: (a) get the dog killed, (b) send the person who has been bitten to the hospital or health centre immediately for vaccine and other treatment;
- if the dog stays healthy, do nothing more;
- if no-one knows the dog, or if the animal which has bitten is a wild one, e.g. hyena or jackal, send the person who has been bitten to the hospital or health centre for vaccine and other treatment.

## How to recognise rabies in a dog

As a rule, rabies in a dog takes one of two forms—dumb or furious.

### Dumb rabies

In dumb rabies, the dog:

- has difficulty in swallowing;
- rarely bites;
- is lethargic (lazy);
- hides;
- dies 3–4 days from a rapid, progressive paralysis.

### Furious rabies

In the early stages of furious rabies, a dog:

- may behave normally for hours at a time;
- is restless;
- hides;
- does not want food, but swallows pieces of wood, straw, stone, etc.
- snaps at everything;
- has spasms in the jaws;
- has spasms in the belly when it tries to eat and drink (these spasms end with a violent effort to breathe, green or bloody frothing liquid comes from its mouth, its eyes become staring and squinting and it paws at its mouth);
- finally, the dog dies within 10 days—its tendency to bite may last until death.

### Treatment

- Once symptoms have developed in a human, there is no treatment.
- Patients with rabies can infect others and should be kept in hospital, well apart from other patients.
- Strict and special barrier nursing is necessary to protect other people, including the health workers caring for him.

# 7. What to Do when Someone has a Belly Pain (Stomach Ache)

When a patient comes to see you because of stomach ache, first ask how bad the pain is.

## If the pain is bad

If the pain came on within a few minutes or hours and the patient has such bad pain that he finds it difficult to walk, and if it is the first time he has had pain like it:

- give a few drops of belladonna (see pharmacopoeia for dosage and method), or an injection of atropine (see pharmacopoeia for dosage);
- send him to hospital or health centre.

If it is not the first time he has had pain like it:

- give a few drops of belladonna (see pharmacopoeia for dosage and method) or an injection of atropine (see pharmacopoeia for dosage);
- see the patient again after 2 hours:
  - if the pain has gone, let the patient go home and tell him to come back if the pain returns;
  - if the pain does come back, send him to the hospital or health centre;
  - if the pain has not gone, send him to the hospital or health centre.

## If the pain is not very bad

If the pain is not very bad and the patient has diarrhoea:

- find out whether he is dehydrated.

Signs of dehydration:

- eyes sunk in the head;
- mouth and tongue dry;
- when you gently pinch the skin, the skinfold remains for a few seconds instead of falling back at once (see Fig. 7.1);
- pulse volume is poor;
- if the patient is less than 8 months old, the fontanelle (the soft spot at the top of the head) is sunken (see Fig. 7.2).

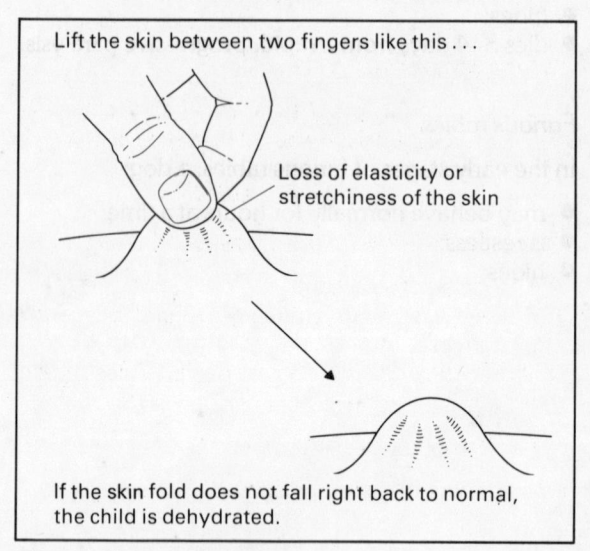

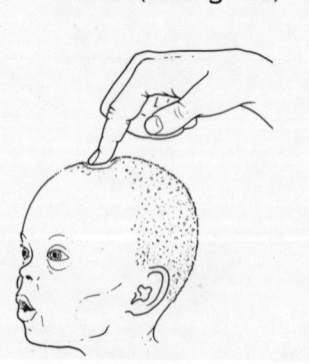

*Lift the skin between two fingers like this...*

*Loss of elasticity or stretchiness of the skin*

*If the skin fold does not fall right back to normal, the child is dehydrated.*

Fig. 7.1  A test for dehydration

*If the soft spot is **sunken**, the baby may be **dehydrated**.*

*If the soft spot is **swollen**, the baby may have **meningitis**.*

Fig. 7.2  Sunken fontanelle

Stomach Pains 41

If these signs are present, the situation is serious. If the patient continues to lose water and salt (through the watery stools of diarrhoea), without having them replaced, he will die.

- send the patient immediately to a hospital or health centre;
- before he leaves, and on the way, he should drink rehydration fluid (see Fig. 7.3).

If the patient is not dehydrated:

- find out if he has a fever;
- find out if there is blood and mucus in his stools.

If these signs are not present:

- tell the patient to eat as usual (if the patient is a child or baby, advise the mother accordingly);
- tell the patient to drink a lot of liquid;
- see the patient on the 3rd day.

If the diarrhoea has stopped by the 3rd day:

- if the patient is an adult:
  - tell him to eat as usual and to stop the rehydration fluid.
- if the patient is a child, give special advice regarding food.

If the diarrhoea has not stopped:

- send the patient to a hospital or health centre.

**Rehydration fluid**

There are many special packets of rehydration salts available in many areas. If you have these:

- into one clean litre bottle put:
  - the contents of 1 packet,
  - one litre of clean water (boiled and cooled if possible).
  (Do not boil the water after putting in the contents of the packet).
- Give this fluid to the patient as long as he is thirsty or one or two cupfuls for every watery stool he passes. Adults will need several litres every day.
  (If there is vomiting, begin by giving sips or spoonfuls of the fluid).
- Show the family how to prepare and use the fluid.
- Leave a few packets with the family.
- Tell the members of the family, as well as the patient, not to use the fluid more than 18–24 hours after it has been made.

If you do not have packets of the special rehydration salts, prepare the following fluid (Fig. 7.3):

- Into a clean 1 litre bottle, put:
- 1 litre of cooled boiled water;
- 2 level tablespoonfuls of sugar or honey;
- ¼ teaspoonful of salt and
- ¼ teaspoonful of bicarbonate of soda.
- Show the family how to make this fluid.
- Supervise them while they make up the mixture, making certain that they have washed their hands first.
- The fluid should taste less salty than tears.

---

**Rehydration drink – to prevent and treat dehydration**

In 1 litre of cooled boiled water    put    2 level tablespoons of sugar or honey (honey is better)    and    ¼ teaspoon salt

and

¼ teaspoon bicarbonate of soda.

If you do not have soda, use another ¼ teaspoon of salt.

If available, add half a cup of orange juice or a little lemon juice to the drink.

---

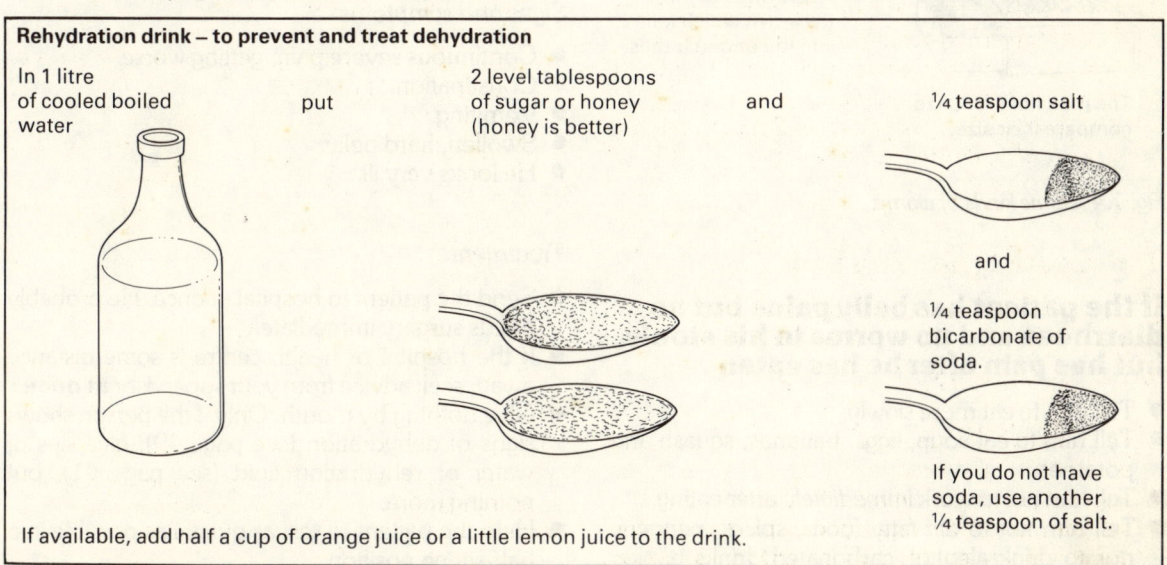

Fig. 7.3 Making up a mixture for dehydration

## If the pain is bad and the patient has worms in his stools

(There are several kinds of worms (see Fig. 7.4).)

If the patient is under 6 years old:

- send him to the hospital or health centre.

If the patient is an adult:

- give piperazine (see pharmacopoeia for dosage and method);
- ask if any others in the family have worms and if so treat them also;
- advise on cleanliness.

Roundworm

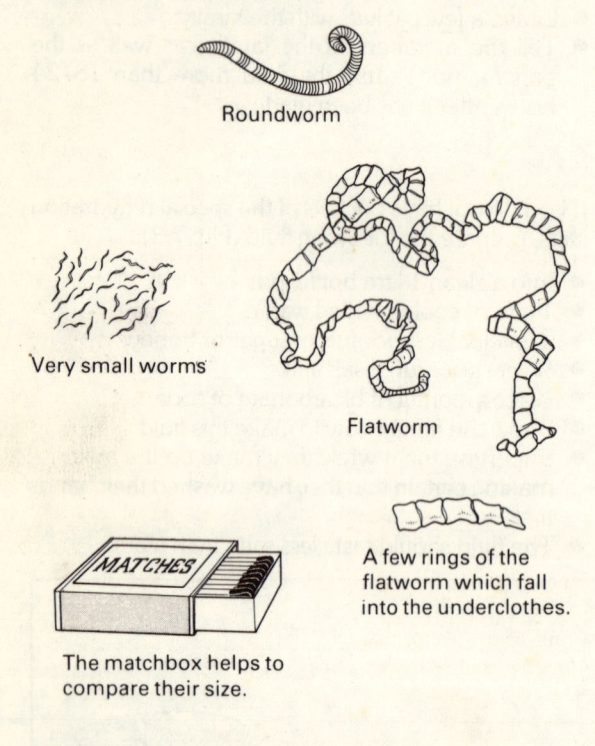

Very small worms

Flatworm

A few rings of the flatworm which fall into the underclothes.

The matchbox helps to compare their size.

*Fig. 7.4 Some kinds of worms*

## If the patient has belly pains but no diarrhoea and no worms in his stools, but has pain after he has eaten

- Tell him to eat more slowly.
- Tell him to eat soup, eggs, bananas, squash and potatoes.
- Tell him not to work *immediately* after eating.
- Tell him not to eat fatty foods, spices, peppers, nor to drink alcohol, carbonated drinks (Coke, pop, etc.) or coffee.

- Give him some drops of belladonna (see pharmacopoeia for dosage) to take for 2 weeks.
- See the patient again in 2 weeks' time.

If, after 2 weeks:

- he is better:
  - tell him to stop taking belladonna;
  - tell him to continue to eat slowly, and to avoid fatty foods.
- he is no better:
  - send him to the hospital or health centre.

## Emergency problems of the gut (acute abdomen)

Acute abdomen is the name given to a number of sudden, severe conditions of the stomach (belly) or gut, for which immediate surgery is often needed to prevent death (Fig. 7.5).

Examples include appendicitis (inflammation of the sac attached to the gut) (Fig. 7.6), peritonitis (inflammation of the lining of the bag that holds the gut) (Fig. 7.7), and gut blockage (Fig. 7.8). The latter may be due to several things, e.g. a ball of roundworms, or a loop of gut which has become pinched, or a bit of gut which has slipped inside the bit of gut below it, and so on.

If a person has continuous severe gut pain with vomiting, but does not have diarrhoea, he is likely to have an acute abdomen.

*Signs and symptoms*

- Continuous severe pain, getting worse.
- Constipation.
- Vomiting.
- Swollen, hard belly.
- He looks very ill.

*Treatment*

- Send the patient to hospital at once. He probably needs surgery immediately.
- If the hospital or health centre is some distance away, seek advice from your supervisor **at once**.
- Give nothing by mouth. Only if the person shows signs of dehydration (see page 40), give sips of water or rehydration fluid (see page 41), but nothing more.
- Help the patient to rest as quietly as possible in a half-sitting position.
- Do **not** give an enema.

## Stomach Pains 43

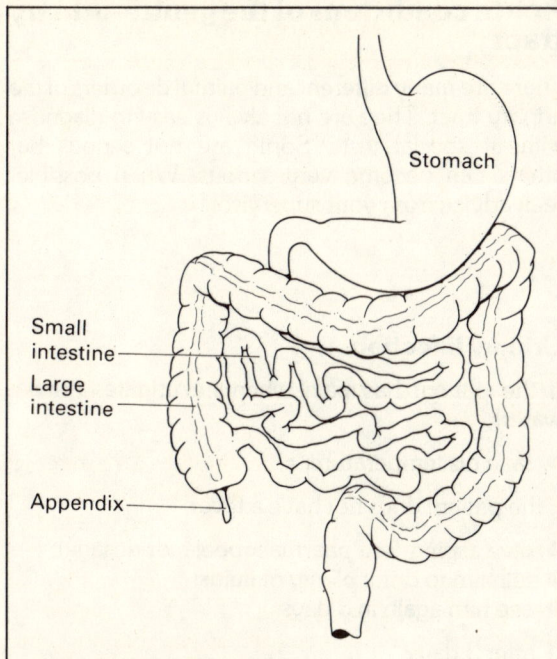

### Appendicitis, Peritonitis

These dangerous conditions often require surgery. Seek medical help fast.

Appendicitis is an infection of the **appendix**, a finger-shaped sac attached to the large intestine in the lower right-hand part of the belly. An infected appendix sometimes bursts open, causing **peritonitis**.

Peritonitis is an acute, serious infection of the lining of the cavity or bag that holds the gut. It results when the appendix or another part of the gut bursts or is torn.

*Fig. 7.5 Appendicitis and peritonitis*

The main sign is a steady pain in the belly that gets worse and worse.

The pain often begins around the navel ('bellybutton'),

but it soon moves to the lower right side.

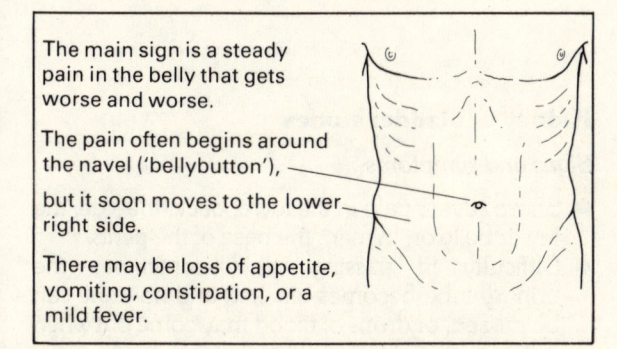

There may be loss of appetite, vomiting, constipation, or a mild fever.

*Fig. 7.6 Signs of appendicitis and areas of pain*

Slowly, but forcefully, press on the abdomen a little above the left groin until it hurts a little.

Then quickly remove the hand.

If a very sharp pain (**rebound pain**) occurs when the hand is removed, appendicitis or peritonitis is likely.

If no rebound pain occurs above the left groin, try the same test above the right groin.

*Fig. 7.7 Method of testing for peritonitis or appendicitis*

Steady, severe pain in the belly.

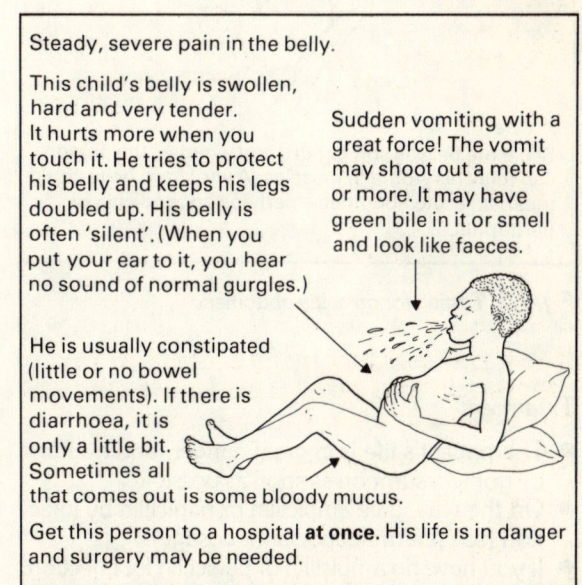

This child's belly is swollen, hard and very tender. It hurts more when you touch it. He tries to protect his belly and keeps his legs doubled up. His belly is often 'silent'. (When you put your ear to it, you hear no sound of normal gurgles.)

Sudden vomiting with a great force! The vomit may shoot out a metre or more. It may have green bile in it or smell and look like faeces.

He is usually constipated (little or no bowel movements). If there is diarrhoea, it is only a little bit. Sometimes all that comes out is some bloody mucus.

Get this person to a hospital **at once**. His life is in danger and surgery may be needed.

*Fig. 7.8 Signs of an obstructed gut*

When peritonitis (inflammation of the tissue in the belly) is severe:

- the abdomen becomes hard like a board;
- the patient feels pain when his belly is touched even very lightly (Fig. 7.9).

First, ask the person to point with one finger where it hurts.

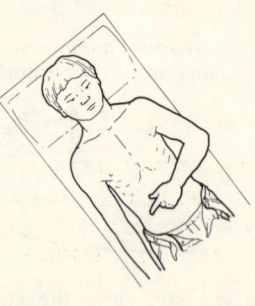

Then, beginning on the opposite side from the spot where he has pointed, press gently on different parts of the belly to see where it hurts most.

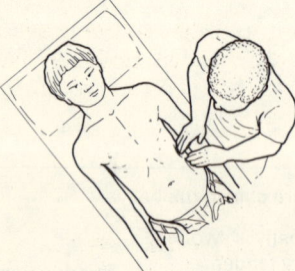

See if the belly is soft or hard and whether the person can relax his stomach muscles. A very hard belly could mean an acute abdomen – perhaps appendicitis or peritonitis.

Fig. 7.9 Testing for an acute abdomen

## Treatment

- The patient's life is in great danger, and he must be got to a surgeon as soon as possible.
- On the way, give ampicillin or penicillin by injection (see pharmacopoeia for dosage).
- If you have no ampicillin or penicillin for injection, give either antibiotic by mouth. Also give chloramphenicol or tetracycline (see pharmacopoeia for dosage) with very little water.

# Acute conditions of the genito-urinary tract

There are many different and painful disorders of the urinary tract. They are not always easy to diagnose without special tests. Some are not serious but others can become very serious. When possible, seek advice from your supervisor.

## Urinary infection

If the patient has pain when he urinates (passes water):

- take his temperature.

If the patient does not have a fever:

- give aspirin (see pharmacopoeia for dosage);
- tell him to drink plenty of fluids;
- see him again in 3 days.

If, after 3 days:

- he is better:
  - tell him to continue to drink plenty of water;
- he is not better:
  - send him to hospital or a health centre.

If the patient has a fever:

- give him sulphadiazine tablets (see pharmacopoeia for dosage);
- see him again after 5 days.

If, after 5 days:

- he is better:
  - tell him to continue to drink more fluid than usual;
- he is not better:
  - send him to hospital or a health centre.

## Kidney or bladder stones

*Signs and symptoms*

- Sharp severe pain in the lower back, the side, the lower belly or, in men, the base of the penis.
- Difficulty in passing urine—sometimes the urinary tube becomes blocked and no urine can be passed, or drops of blood may come out when the person tries to pass urine.
- Fever if the urine is infected.

*Treatment*

- Fluids and antibiotics as for infection (see above).
- Give aspirin or other pain-killer.
- Give an anti-spasmodic medicine (see pharmacopoeia).
- Tell the patient to try to pass water whilst lying down (this sometimes helps the stone in the bladder to roll back and so free the opening to the urinary tube).
- If this does not help, get medical advice. Surgery may be needed.

**Enlarged prostate gland**

This is common in older men. It is caused by the swelling of the gland which lies between the urinary bladder and the urinary tube (urethra).

*Signs and symptoms*

- The patient has difficulty in passing urine and maybe in passing stools also. The urine may dribble, drip, or the opening may have become blocked completely and the patient may not have been able to pass urine for many hours.
- Fever, if the urine has become infected.
- The patient may be sleepy or confused.

*Treatment*

- Seek advice immediately. Surgery may be needed.
- Help the patient to sit in a bath of hot (not very hot) water; this sometimes helps to pass urine.
- If there is fever, begin a course of ampicillin or tetracycline (see pharmacopoeia for dosage).
- If medical help is not available, it may be necessary to pass a catheter.

*Using a catheter*

- **Never use a catheter unless it is absolutely necessary and it is impossible to get medical help in time.** Even careful use of a catheter sometimes causes dangerous infections or damages the urinary canal.
- If any urine **at all** is being passed, do not use the catheter.
- Try the hot bath treatment (above).
- Begin the course of antibiotics (see above).
- Only if the patient has a very full or a very painful bladder, and cannot urinate at all, or if he shows signs of poisoning (is drowsy, sleepy or confused) should the catheter be passed.

*Signs and symptoms of urinary poisoning*

- The breath smells like urine.
- Feet and face are swollen.
- Confusion, drowsiness.
- Vomiting.

*How to pass a catheter* (Fig. 7.10)

If the patient shows signs of urine poisoning, do not let all the urine come out at once. Let it out slowly, over a period of 1–2 hours.

Women sometimes have trouble urinating after giving birth and need a catheter put in. The method is similar, but the woman's urinary tube is much shorter.

**Gonorrhoea (a venereal disease)**

It is important to distinguish between an enlarged prostate and gonorrhoea. Both can make it difficult to pass urine and in a young man the cause is likely to be gonorrhoea.

*Signs and symptoms*

- Pain with passing water (at first).
- Drops of pus from the penis.
- Fever (sometimes).
- Difficulty in passing water or no water is passed.

*Treatment*

- Encourage the passing of water (as described above).
- Get medical advice.
- Begin a course of penicillin (see pharmacopoeia for dosage).
- Pass a catheter if advised to do so by your supervisor.
- See that everyone who has had sex with the man is seen and also treated for gonorrhoea if necessary.
- Boil or sterilise all equipment, towels, etc. you have used while treating the patient and his sexual associates.

46    First Aid

1. Boil the catheter for 15 minutes.

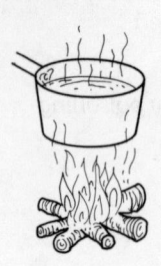

2. Wash the penis and the whole area around it well with soap and warm water.

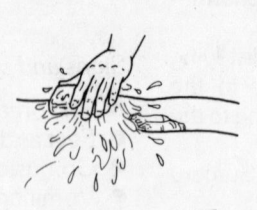

3. Wash your hands with boiled water and soap.

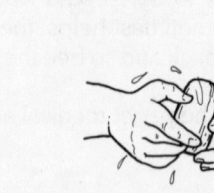

4. Cover the area around the penis with a very clean cloth, sterilized if possible.

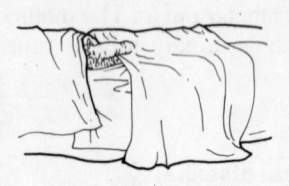

5. Wash your hands with alcohol. (If you have sterile gloves, use them.)

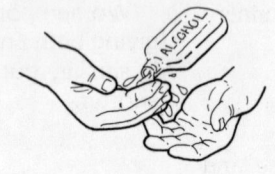

6. Lubricate the catheter with antibiotic ointment or a sterile lubricant.

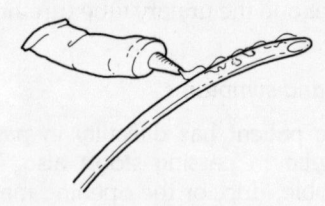

7. Insert the catheter little by little, very carefully.

If the catheter does not go in easily, roll it gently between your fingers and move the penis, but **never force the catheter**. It is very easy to injure the urinary canal and cause serious problems. When urine starts to come out, do not try to push the catheter in any more.

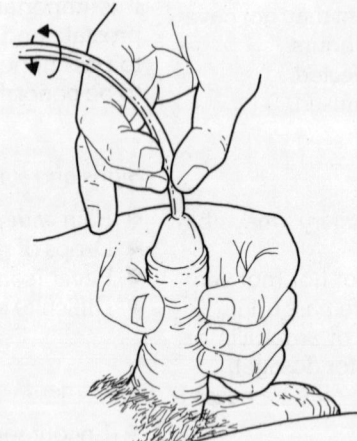

BE VERY CAREFUL THAT THE CATHETER NEVER TOUCHES ANYTHING BUT THE OPENING OF THE PENIS AND YOUR HANDS.

Keep the penis in this position so that the urine canal is not bent.

Fig. 7.10 *How to use a catheter*

# 8. What to Do when a Pregnant Woman Becomes Ill

## Avoiding illness during pregnancy

As a health worker you are in a position to give advice to pregnant women. Briefly, you should teach them:

- how important it is to eat well;
- that it is good to use a little iodised salt in their food each day (but not *too* much as this can cause swelling of the feet and other problems);
- how important it is to keep clean—not only to bathe or wash regularly, but also to keep their hair and teeth clean;
- that they should avoid taking medicines but vitamin and iron pills, in the right dosages, can be good—aspirin or antacids may be taken occasionally;
- that they should not smoke or drink alcoholic substances during pregnancy;
- that they should continue to work and take exercise, but not get too tired;
- that they must keep away from children with measles, especially German measles (rubella);
- that it is best to avoid sexual contact during the last month of pregnancy as this may break the bag of waters and cause infection.

If, in spite of taking your good advice, a pregnant woman becomes ill, it is important to be able to tell which conditions you can treat and which conditions are dangerous and require medical attention.

## Some minor discomforts and difficulties

### Nausea and vomiting

This is often worse in the morning during the second and third months of pregnancy. It helps to eat and drink something before getting out of bed. It is also better to eat small meals often, rather than large amounts of food. Greasy food should not be taken.

### Burning or pain in the pit of the stomach (acid indigestion and heartburn)

Again, it helps to eat only small amounts of food at a time. Eating papaya or paw-paw also helps to aid digestion. If appropriate, encourage the woman to drink milk. Suggest she sleeps with her head and chest raised.

### Swelling of the feet

This usually occurs during the last months of pregnancy and is caused by pressure of the child in the woman's womb (uterus) (Fig. 8.1).

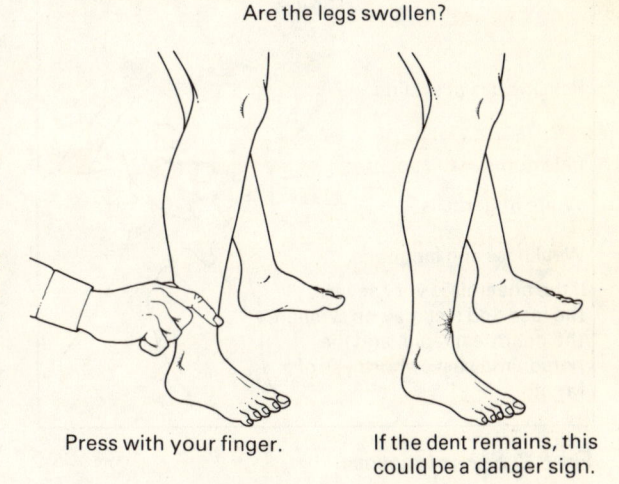

Are the legs swollen?

Press with your finger. If the dent remains, this could be a danger sign.

*Fig. 8.1 Testing for swelling of the feet and ankles*

It is more likely to happen if the woman is anaemic, malnourished or if she eats too much salt. She should rest at various times of the day, eat more nutritious food with less salt and drink tea made from corn (maize) silk. (Boil a handful of cornsilk in a medium-sized pan of water and drink one or two glasses each day.)

## Anaemia and malnutrition

Many women are anaemic even before they become pregnant, and by nourishing the fetus, they become even more anaemic during pregnancy (Fig. 8.2). If the woman is to produce a healthy baby she must eat foods rich in protein and iron. These include beans, groundnuts, chicken, milk, cheese, eggs, insects, meat, fish, and dark green leafy vegetables. If it is difficult to get enough nutritious food, she should take iron and vitamin pills in proper doses. These will strengthen her blood and help to prevent dangerous bleeding after the birth of her baby. If possible, the iron pills should contain folic acid and vitamic C.

If the woman's hands and face are also swollen, get medical advice.

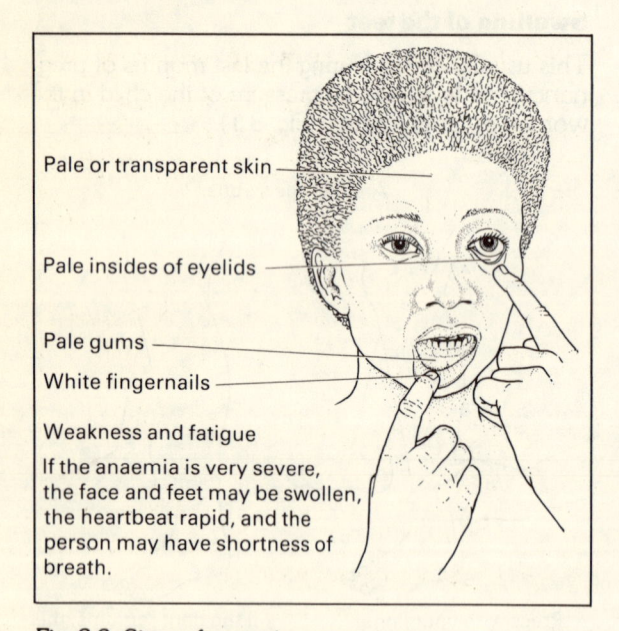

Pale or transparent skin
Pale insides of eyelids
Pale gums
White fingernails
Weakness and fatigue
If the anaemia is very severe, the face and feet may be swollen, the heartbeat rapid, and the person may have shortness of breath.

*Fig. 8.2 Signs of anaemia*

## Low back pain

Low back pain is very common in pregnancy. It can be helped by taking care to stand and sit with the back straight and by doing back-bending exercises each morning. The woman should also be told to sleep on a firm flat surface at night. (See Fig. 8.3).

Always standing straight

Like this    Not like this

Sleep on a firm flat surface

Like this

Not like this

Do back-bending exercises like this

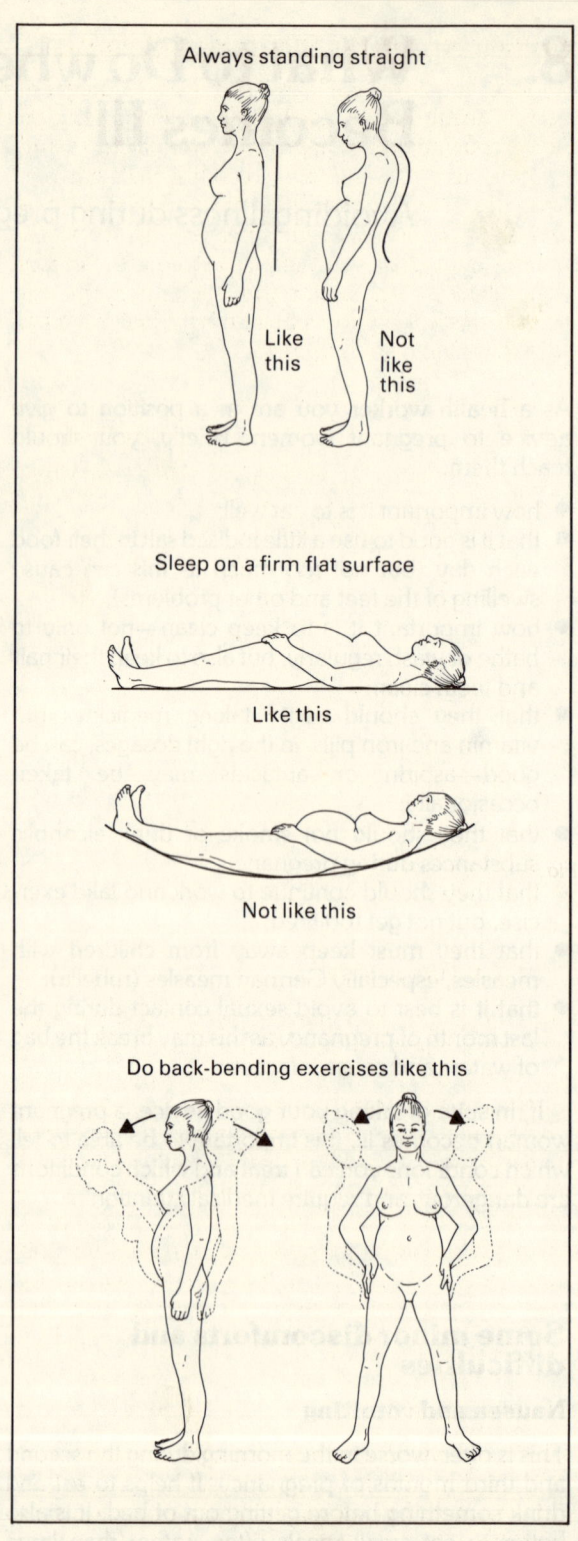

*Fig. 8.3 Good practices for a pregnant woman*

Illness During Pregnancy 49

### Swollen veins in the legs (varicose veins)

Swollen leg veins are fairly common in pregnant women and are due to the baby's weight pressing on the veins in the groin. The woman should be advised to spend less time standing or sitting with her feet down. If she has no choice but to stand or sit for long periods, she should lie with her feet up for a few minutes every half-hour and also sleep with her feet higher than the rest of her body. Wrapping the legs with an elastic bandage may also help, but this must be taken off at night (Fig. 8.4).

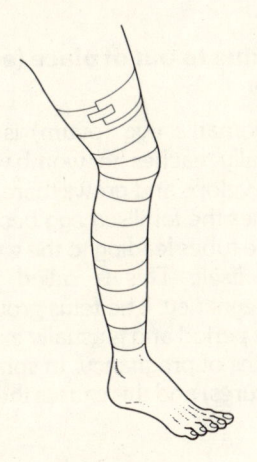

*Fig. 8.4 Bandaging for varicose veins*

### Piles (haemorrhoids)

Piles or haemorrhoids are varicose veins of the anus or rectum, which feel like small lumps. They may be painful but are not dangerous. Often they go away after the baby is born.

They are often caused by constipation and the woman should be advised to eat plenty of fruit and food with fibre such as cassava or bran.

Certain bitter plant juices such as those from cactus plants, witch hazel, etc. dabbed on the piles often help to shrink them. Pain can sometimes be relieved by kneeling face downwards with the buttocks in the air and elbows on the floor (Fig. 8.5).

### Constipation

If the pregnant woman has constipation she should be advised to drink lots of clean water, to eat fruit and food with fibre such as cassava and to take more exercise.

Strong laxatives should **not** be taken.

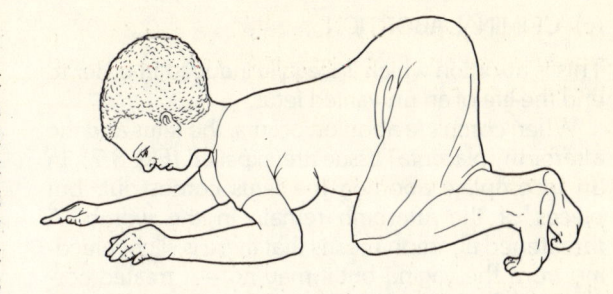

*Fig. 8.5 Position to relieve pain from piles*

## Danger signs in pregnant women

If, in spite of all care and advice, any of the following happens, medical help should be obtained at once.

### Bleeding

If a pregnant woman loses any amount of blood—however little—from the birth-opening (vagina), she should be treated as an emergency.

*Vaginal bleeding due to abortion (miscarriage)*

Abortion is expulsion of the fetus from the womb during the first 20 weeks of pregnancy (Fig. 8.6).

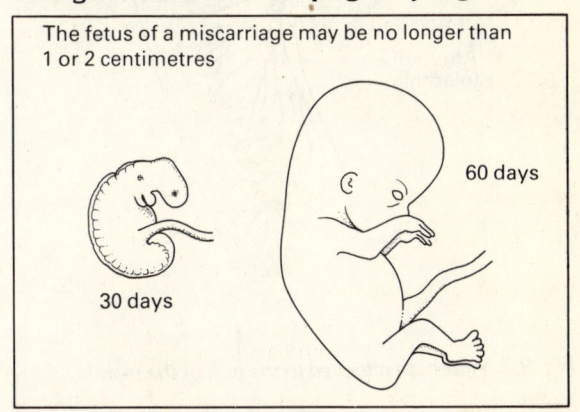

The fetus of a miscarriage may be no longer than 1 or 2 centimetres

30 days

60 days

*Fig. 8.6 The fetus of a miscarriage*

There are three kinds of abortion:

(a) SPONTANEOUS ABORTION

This is loss of the unborn fetus during the first 3 months of pregnancy.

(b) THERAPEUTIC ABORTION

This is abortion which is legally induced by drugs in order to save the woman's life.

## (c) CRIMINAL ABORTION

This is abortion which is illegally induced in order to end the life of an unwanted fetus.

When complete abortion occurs, the fetus and the afterbirth (placenta) tissue are expelled (Fig. 8.7). In an incomplete abortion the fetus comes out, but pieces of the afterbirth remain in the womb. A threatened abortion means that there is slight bleeding from the vagina but it may not—if treated correctly and quickly—result in abortion. The woman should stay in bed until the bleeding has stopped for 2 days.

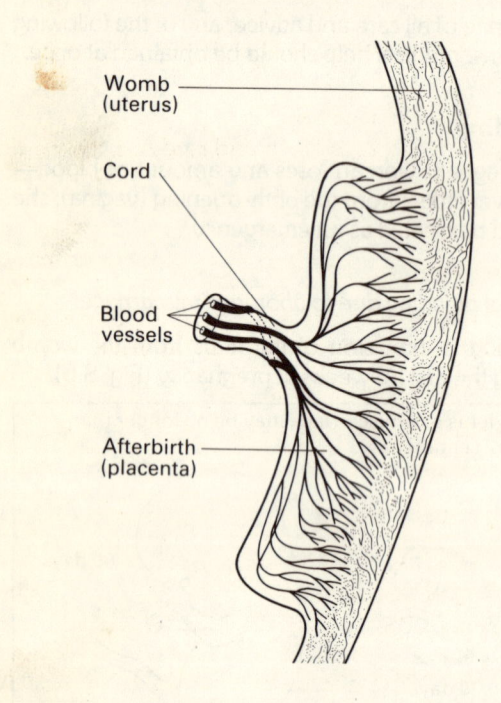

*Fig. 8.7 Afterbirth attached to the wall of the womb*

*Signs and symptoms of miscarriage or abortion*

- Bleeding: either slight or severe.
- Rapid pulse rate.
- Low back pain.
- Belly pain.
- Belly distension.
- Shock: depending upon the amount of blood loss.
- Sometimes vomiting.

*Treatment*

- Care for shock (see page 6).
- Transfer the woman carefully and gently to medical help—preferably to a hospital.

Meanwhile:

- keep the woman quiet and calm;
- observe and record pulse and respiration rates;
- collect any tissue or clotted blood which may be discharged from the womb.

## Bleeding due to out of place (ectopic) pregnancy

When a woman's egg (ovum) is fertilised by her man, it usually reaches her womb within 2 days, and the fetus develops and grows there.

Sometimes the fertilised egg becomes embedded in one of the tubes leading to the womb instead of in the womb itself. This is called 'out-of-place' or 'ectopic' pregnancy. The fetus grows in the tube for only a short period and is usually expelled during the first 3 months of pregnancy. In some cases the tube bursts (ruptures) and this causes the woman to bleed internally.

*Signs and symptoms*

- Sudden acute belly pain radiating to the shoulder.
- Tender belly.
- Nausea and vomiting.
- Weak, rapid pulse.
- Pale, cold, moist skin.
- Sweating.

If the temperature and blood pressure are taken, these will be found to be low.

*Treatment*

- Arrange for transfer to hospital or medical aid immediately.

Meanwhile:

- care for shock;
- keep the woman's head level with the rest of her body;
- calm and reassure the woman;
- observe and record pulse and respiration rates;
- begin artificial respiration and cardiac massage immediately if the woman collapses (see page 14).

## Vaginal bleeding late in pregnancy (during the last weeks)

Vaginal bleeding which occurs during the last weeks of pregnancy (Fig. 8.8) is extremely dangerous and can result in the deaths of both woman and baby. It means that the afterbirth (placenta) is blocking the birth opening.

*Signs and symptoms*

- Bleeding.
- Severe shock.

*Treatment*

- Arrange for transfer to hospital or medical aid immediately.

Meanwhile:

- treat for shock (see page 6);
- begin artificial respiration and cardiac massage if necessary.

## Severe anaemia

In cases of severe anaemia, the patient will have the following signs and symptoms (see Fig. 8.2):

- pale or transparent-looking skin;
- pale insides of eyelids;
- pale gums;
- white fingernails;
- weakness and tiredness;
- swelling of face and feet;
- rapid pulse rate;
- shortness of breath.

A poor diet, hookworms, chronic diarrhoea, dysentery and malaria all cause anaemia. If any of these are present they should be treated, as well as the anaemia. If severe anaemia is left untreated the woman may die from blood loss at childbirth. A good diet is not enough to correct the condition in time, and iron tablets should be given. Seek medical advice. If possible, the woman should have her baby in hospital because she may need extra blood.

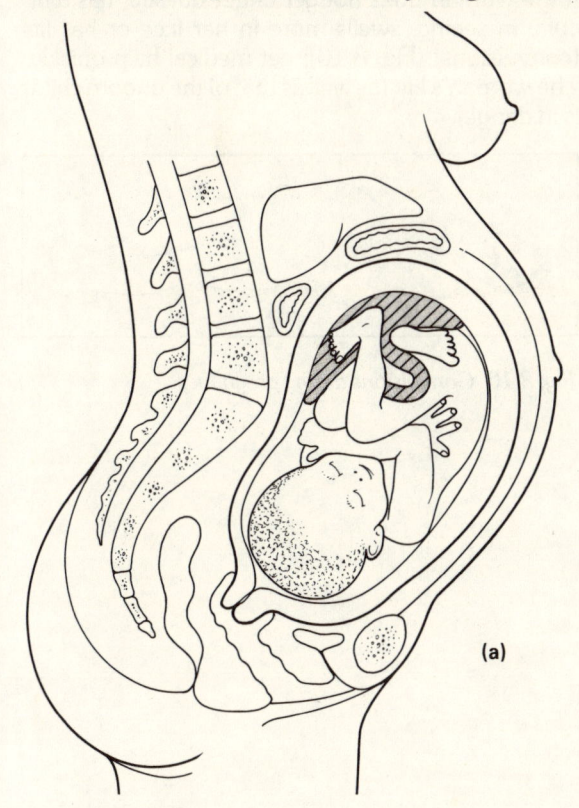

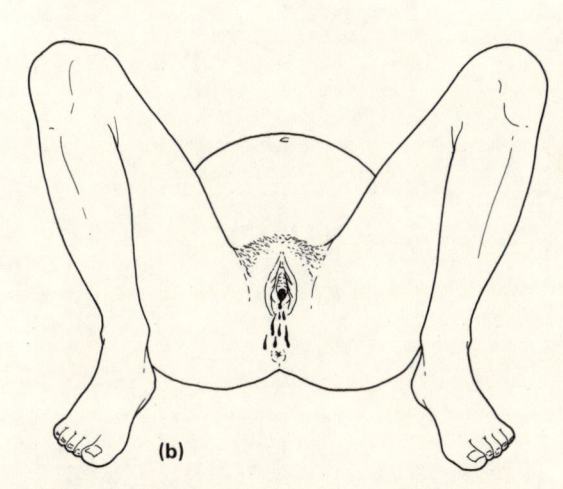

*Fig. 8.8 Signs of a miscarriage. (a) The position of the baby in its mother's belly towards the end of pregnancy is normal but (b) the woman is losing blood through the vagina.*

## Swelling

Swelling of the feet, hands and face with dizziness and sometimes blurred vision are signs of poisoning

52  First Aid

of pregnancy (toxaemia) (Fig. 8.9). If you have the equipment and know how to do so, check for weight-gain, check blood pressure and the amount of protein in the woman's urine.

**During the last 3 months of pregnancy:**

the woman has headaches or trouble seeing

and

her face and hands begin to swell,

she may be suffering from

**TOXAEMIA OF PREGNANCY**

If only her feet swell, it probably is not serious. But watch out for other signs of toxaemia.

Use little or no salt.

**GET MEDICAL HELP!**

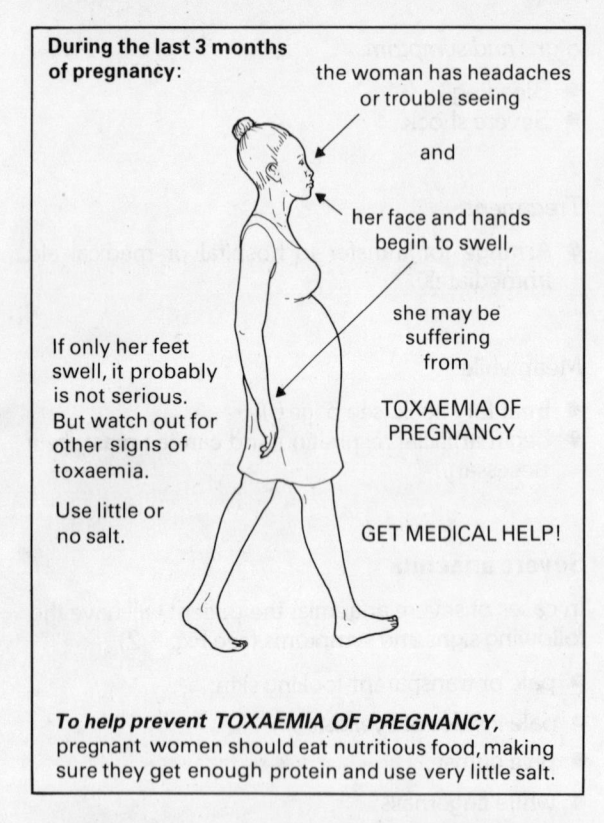

**To help prevent TOXAEMIA OF PREGNANCY,** pregnant women should eat nutritious food, making sure they get enough protein and use very little salt.

*Fig. 8.9  Signs and symptoms of poisoning (toxaemia) of pregnancy*

*Treatment*
- Quiet rest in bed.
- No salt in or with food.

If the woman does not get better quickly, has difficulty in seeing, swells more in her face or has fits (convulsions) (Fig. 8.10), get medical help quickly. The woman's life (as well as that of the unborn child) is in danger.

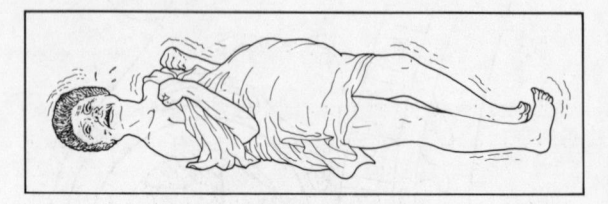

*Fig. 8.10  Convulsions during pregnancy*

# 9. What to Do when a Pregnant Woman Goes into Labour

Birth is, of course, a natural event. If the mother is healthy and there are no complications, the baby can be born without help from anyone. In fact, during a normal birth the less everyone does the better.

Difficulties do occur in childbirth, however, and sometimes the life of the mother or child, or both, may be in danger. If you think that a birth may be difficult or dangerous, a skilled midwife or experienced doctor should be contacted at once.

## Signs of special risk

- If the woman begins to bleed before labour.
- If the woman has signs of toxaemia of pregnancy (see page 52).
- If the woman is suffering from a chronic or an acute illness such as diabetes, or a heart condition.
- If the woman is very anaemic.
- If the woman has had trouble or severe bleeding during previous births.
- If the woman is going to have twins.
- If the woman is very short or has very narrow hips.
- If the woman is under 15, over 40 or is having her first baby at the age of 35 or more.
- If the baby is not in a normal position in the womb (see Figs 9.1, 9.2, 9.3, 9.4).
- If the bag of waters breaks but the woman does not begin labour within a few hours.

For women with any one of these conditions, obtain midwifery or medical help.

## The stages of labour

There are three stages of labour.

(1) The first stage lasts from the beginning of strong sudden tightenings of the womb (contractions) until the baby drops down into the birth canal (vagina).

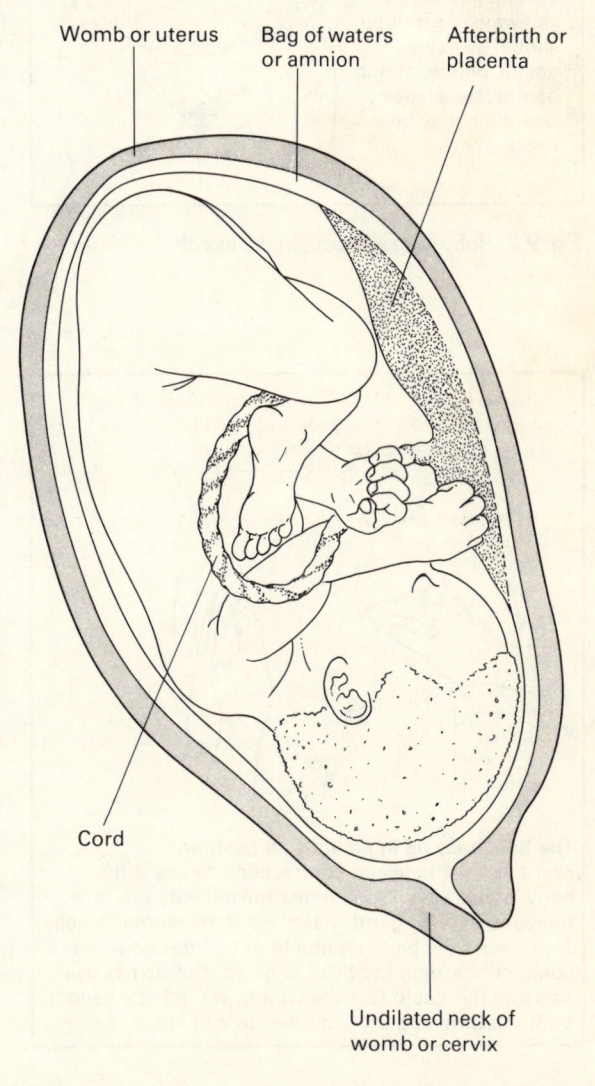

*Fig. 9.1 Normal position of the fetus in the womb (uterus)*

(2) The second stage lasts from the dropping of the baby into the vagina until it is born.
(3) The third stage lasts from the birth of the baby until the afterbirth (placenta) comes out.

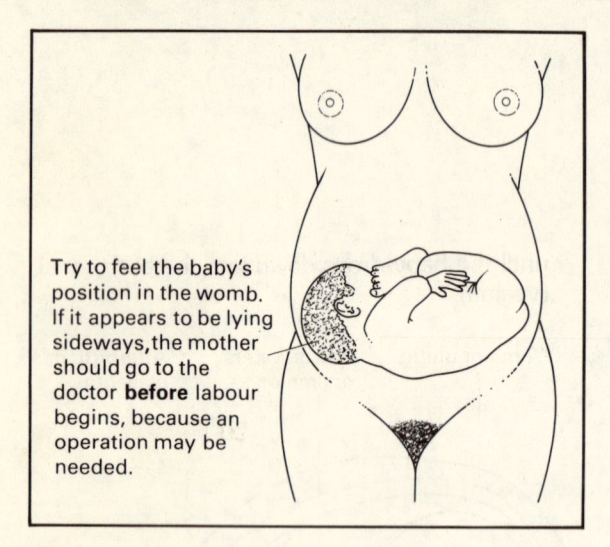

Try to feel the baby's position in the womb. If it appears to be lying sideways, the mother should go to the doctor **before** labour begins, because an operation may be needed.

*Fig. 9.2 Baby lying sideways in the womb*

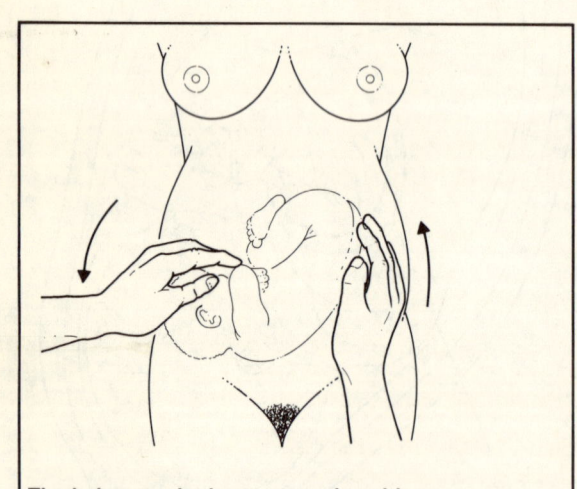

**The baby may be in an unusual position.** Feel the belly between contractions to see if the baby is **sideways**. Sometimes the midwife can turn the baby through **gentle** handling of the woman's belly. Try to work the baby around little by little between contractions, until the head is down. But **do not use force** as this could tear the womb. If the baby cannot be turned, try to get the mother to a hospital.

*Fig. 9.3 Turning the baby in the womb*

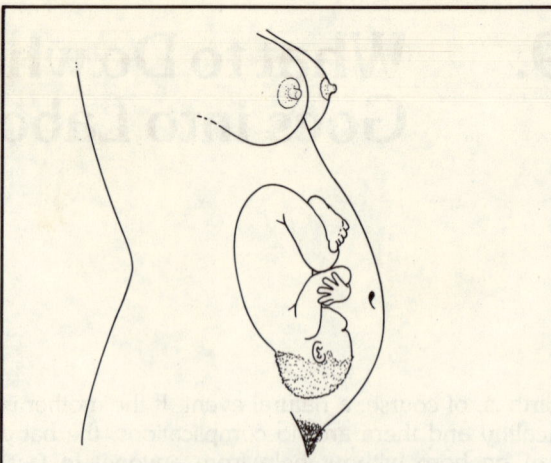

**If the baby is facing forward** rather than backward, you may feel the lumpy arms and legs rather than the rounded back. This is usually no big problem, but labour may be longer and cause the woman more back pain. She should change position often, as this may help to turn the baby.

*Fig. 9.4 Baby facing forward in the womb*

Whilst delivery is not a disease, the accidents which may occur during delivery may be dangerous for the mother and child. Delivery should therefore be supervised.

You should tell the people who attend deliveries:

- to keep their hands clean;
- to use clean towels (or pieces of material);
- to use clean instruments (e.g. scissors or razor blade);
- to use only clean water (boiled if possible);
- to keep the woman and baby clean;
- to send for you at once if there is any difficulty.

## How to see whether the woman is about to have her baby

Usually the woman is 9 months pregnant (Fig. 9.5), although sometimes (but rarely) 7–8 months pregnant and she starts to have pains every 5–10 minutes either in the lower belly or in the lower part of her back. During these pains her womb becomes hard.

A little pink fluid or blood comes out of the vagina.

At the beginning of her delivery, the woman sometimes loses a large quantity of water, 'the waters' (it is the water in which the baby has been living while in its mother's belly) and the pains will begin shortly afterwards.

*Pregnant Woman in Labour* 55

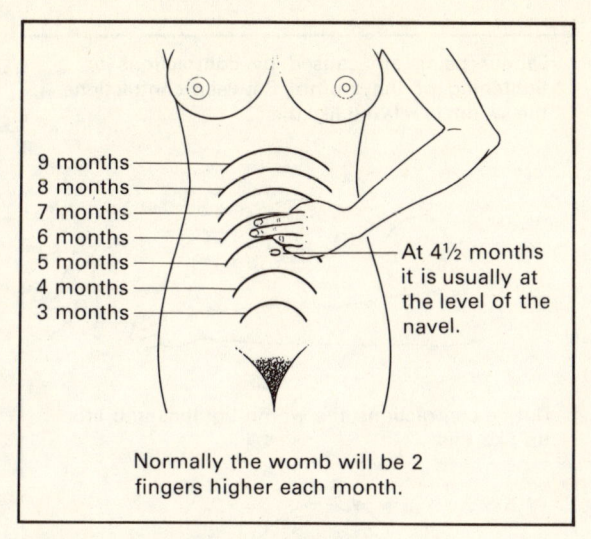

9 months
8 months
7 months
6 months
5 months
4 months
3 months

At 4½ months it is usually at the level of the navel.

Normally the womb will be 2 fingers higher each month.

*Fig. 9.5 Normal growth of the fetus*

## What to do before the baby comes out

- If the woman is frightened, reassure her and ask her to be patient.
- Do not allow more than two people to remain in the room and, if possible, ask them to prepare clean boiled water for washing the mother and baby.
- Ask the woman to pass water (Fig. 9.6).
- Place towels, sheets, smoked banana leaves or newspaper under the woman.
- Wash your hands and forearms with soap and water (Fig. 9.7).
- Wash the woman's genitals.
- Wash your hands and forearms again.
- If the woman says that her waters have already broken, ask her to either squat or lie down until the baby is born (either position is considered safe).
- Do not leave the woman if the pains are severe and when they occur every 2 minutes.
- If the pains become irregular, less strong or less frequent during the first 15–20 hours, send the woman to hospital or a health centre if possible. If not, get medical advice.

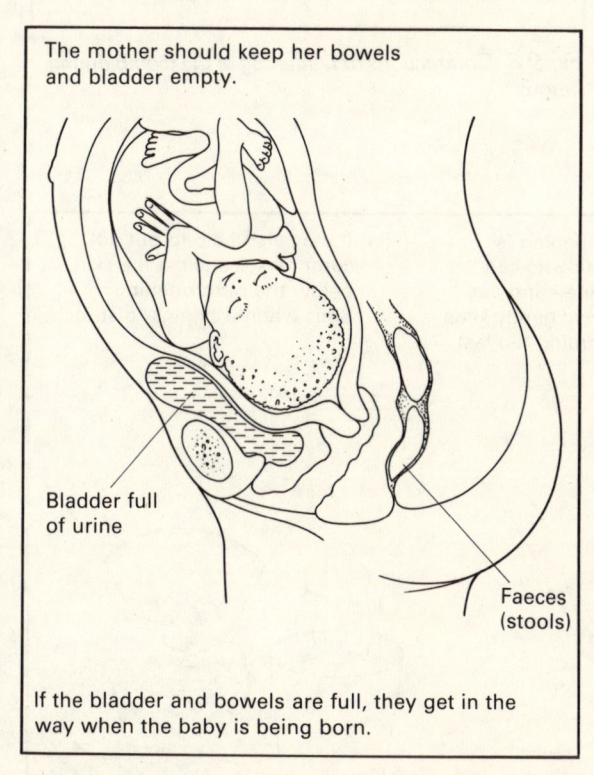

The mother should keep her bowels and bladder empty.

Bladder full of urine

Faeces (stools)

If the bladder and bowels are full, they get in the way when the baby is being born.

*Fig. 9.6 Effect of the mother's full gut and bladder on the birth of a baby*

Wash your hands and forearms with soap and water

then, wash the woman's genitals as well . . . and wash your hands once again.

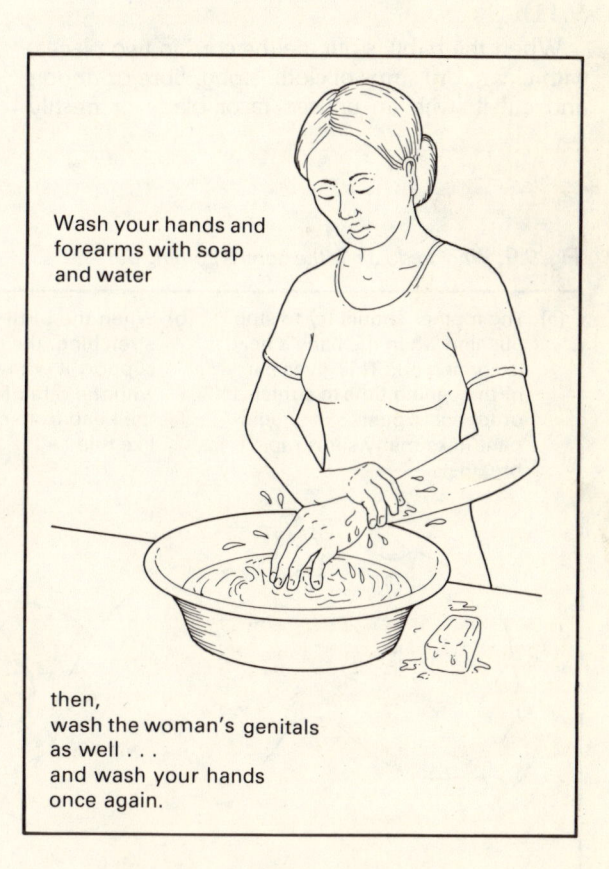

*Fig. 9.7 What to do before the baby is born*

56  First Aid

## What to do while the baby is coming out

When the pains occur every 2 or 3 minutes (Fig. 9.8) and the woman feels a need to push, uncover her genitals and look between her legs, *when she feels the pains.*

*If the head appears* at the opening, as happens in the great majority of deliveries, you will see some hair. To make the baby come out, tell the woman to push every time she feels the pains and to stop pushing when she does not have the pain (see Figs 9.9 and 9.10). After she has pushed several times you will see that the head stays at the opening when the pains stop. From that time onwards, every time the woman feels the pains and begins to push, put your left hand (if you are right-handed) on the baby's head to prevent it from coming out too quickly (If the baby comes out too quickly it may tear the mother's genitals.) Hook your right hand against the woman's body where the baby's face is going to appear.

Once the baby's head is out, the shoulders and the rest of the body are likely to come out easily (Fig. 9.11).

When the baby is out, tie the cord in two places, with clean, dry strips of cloth, string, fibre or ribbon and cut it (with an unused razor blade or freshly

Labour pains are caused by contractions or tightening of the womb. Between contractions, the womb is relaxed like this:

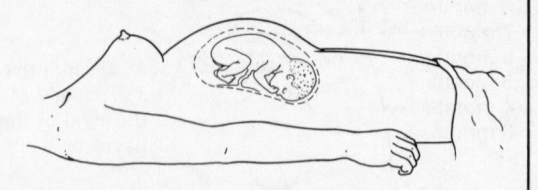

During contractions, the womb tightens and lifts up like this:

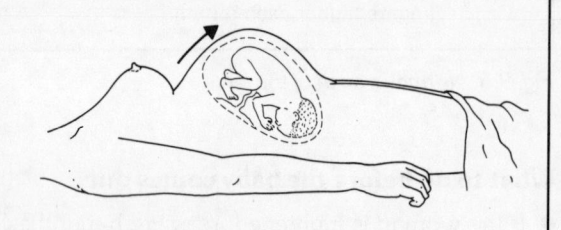

The contractions cause the **cervix** or 'door of the womb' to open – a little more each time.

Fig. 9.8 Contractions or tightening of the womb during labour

Fig. 9.9 What to do while the baby is coming out

(a) The mother should try to stop pushing when the baby's head is coming out: This gives her birth opening time to stretch. In order not to push, she should pant (take many short rapid breaths).

(b) When the birth opening is stretching, the midwife can support it with one hand and with the other hand gently keep the head from coming too fast, like this :

(c) It may also help to put hot compresses against the skin below the birth opening. Start when it begins to stretch.

Pregnant Woman in Labour 57

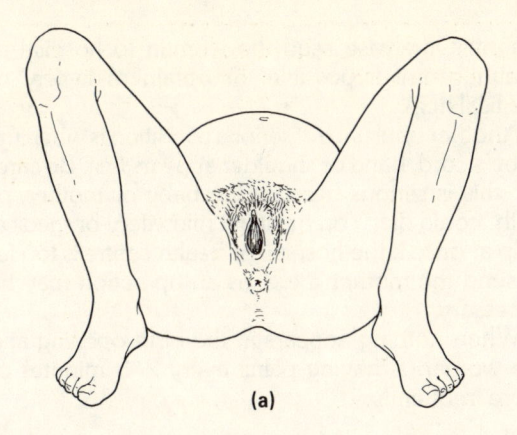

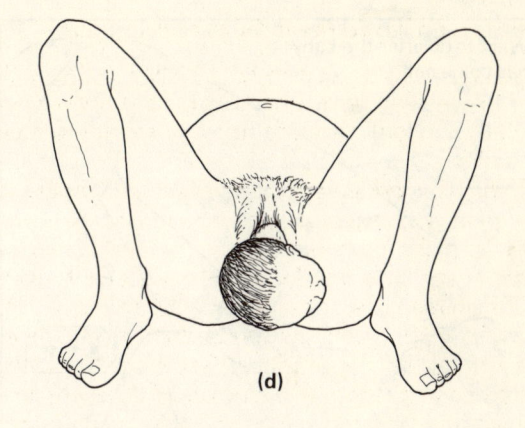

*Fig. 9.10 Stages of labour*

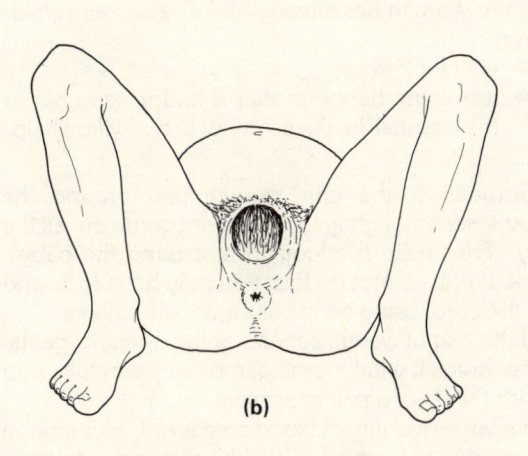

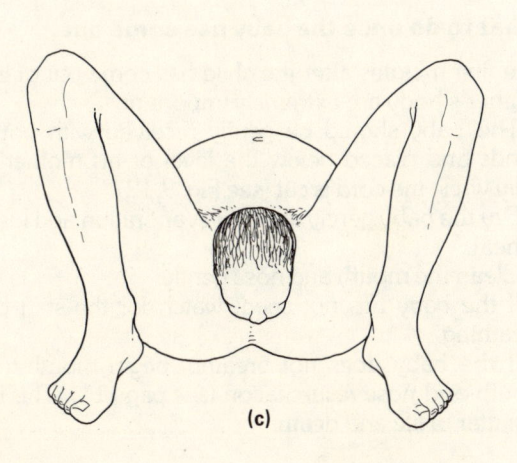

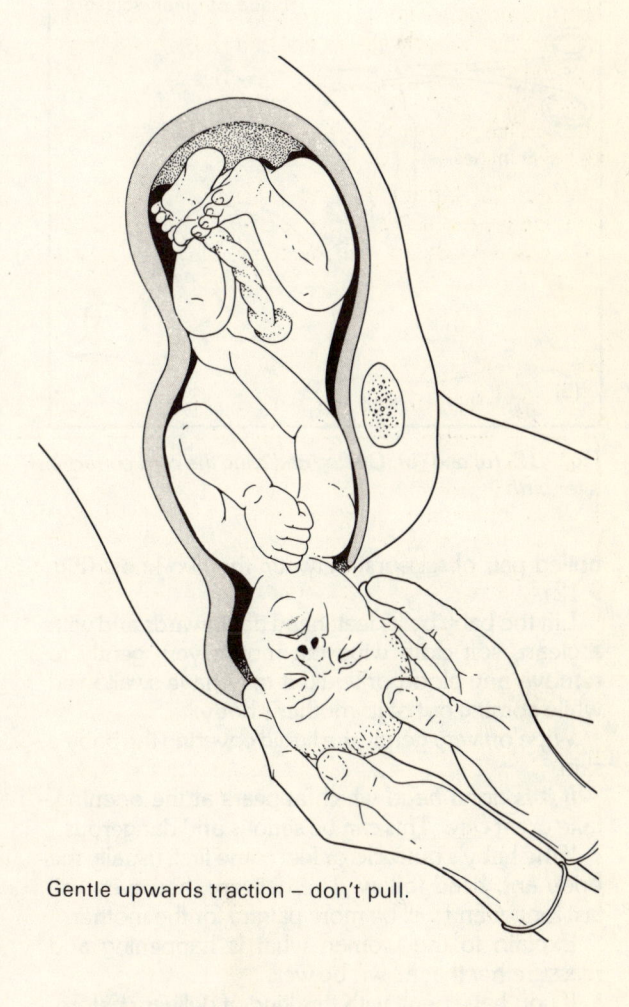

Gentle upwards traction – don't pull.

*Fig. 9.11 Birth of a baby*

58  *First Aid*

**What to do after the baby has come out**

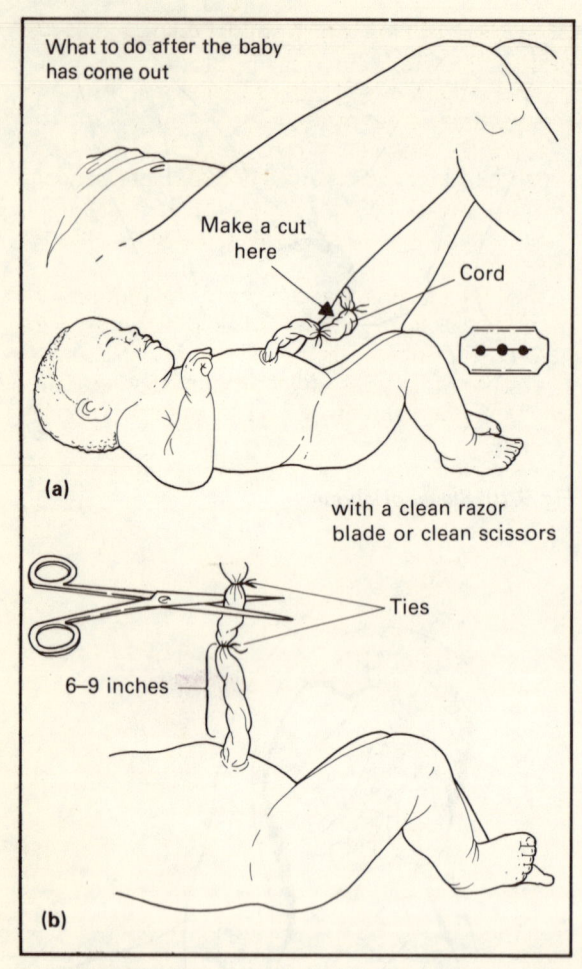

Make a cut here
Cord
(a)
with a clean razor blade or clean scissors
Ties
6–9 inches
(b)

*Fig. 9.12 (a) and (b). Cutting and tying the cord correctly after birth*

boiled pair of scissors) between the two knots (Fig. 9.12).

Lift the baby by its feet, head downwards and with a clean, soft cloth wipe the mouth very gently to remove any blood or liquid it may have swallowed while coming out of its mother's body.

Wipe off very gently the liquid covering the baby's skin.

*If it is not a head* which appears at the opening, take great care. This can be serious and dangerous.

If the baby's buttocks or feet come first, usually the body and head follow. The delivery, however, will last longer and will be more painful for the mother.

Explain to the woman what is happening and reassure her that all will be well.

If you have dealt with this kind of delivery before, and know what to do, act in the way you have been taught. Otherwise send the woman to hospital or health centre if possible, or obtain midwifery or medical help.

Another unusual but serious condition is when the baby's cord, hand or shoulder appears first. Be careful: this is serious because the baby or mother, or both, could die. You must get midwifery or medical help at once if the hospital or health centre is too far to send the mother there, as an operation may be necessary.

When nothing appears at the birth opening and the woman is having pains every 2–3 minutes or more frequently:

- if the woman is giving birth for the first time and the pains are not too severe:
  - wait for 1 hour;
  - if nothing happens after 1 hour, send her to hospital/health centre, or to midwifery help;
- if the woman has already had one or more children:
  - wait for 2 hours;
  - if nothing happens after 2 hours, send her to the hospital/health centre or to midwifery help.

Sometimes the cord is wrapped around the baby's neck so tightly that it cannot come out all the way. Try to slip the loop from around the baby's neck. If you cannot do this, you may have to tie and cut the cord, using boiled blunt-tipped scissors.

If the bag of waters appears at the opening, gently either break it with your finger, or very carefully snip it with the *tip* of a pair of scissors.

If a large quantity of blood comes out, accompany the woman to hospital or health centre on a stretcher and give plenty of warm fluids on the way.

## What to do once the baby has come out

The first minutes after the child has come out of its mother's body are extremely important.

The baby should be gently received with both hands and placed below the level of his mother's belly while the cord is cut (see Fig. 9.12).

Dry the baby gently to avoid evaporation and loss of heat.

Clean the mouth and nose gently.

If the baby has not cried, watch for the start of breathing.

If the baby does not breathe, begin mouth-to-mouth-and-nose resuscitation (see page 11). This is a matter of life and death.

Place a little aureomycin ointment in each eye to prevent infection.

Place the child in close contact with its mother's breast. Her belly will contract, helping the afterbirth to come away and stopping or lessening any bleeding after the delivery.

If the baby begins to suck, 'good' breast feeding will soon be established and this first milk will help to protect the baby from infection and increase love bonding with its mother.

About 15 minutes after the baby's birth, the mother may feel mild pain in her lower belly. This is normal. It is because the afterbirth (placenta) which connected the baby to its mother inside her womb is coming out. After a few minutes of these pains, the afterbirth will appear in the vaginal opening. It is a large piece of flesh which should come out in one piece.

Do not pull the cord because it may tear. Wait until the placenta comes out by itself.

Once the placenta is out, go back to the baby. Wash him and clean his eyes. Put a light bandage over the place where the cord was (Fig. 9.13).

Return to the mother to check that all the placenta has come out.

If all the placenta has not come out an hour after the birth, or if the mother is losing blood from the vagina, gently massage the top part of her womb, or if you have it, give an intramuscular injection of oxytocin (the contents of a 5 I.U. ampoule) into her buttock.

If the placenta has not come out 2 hours after the

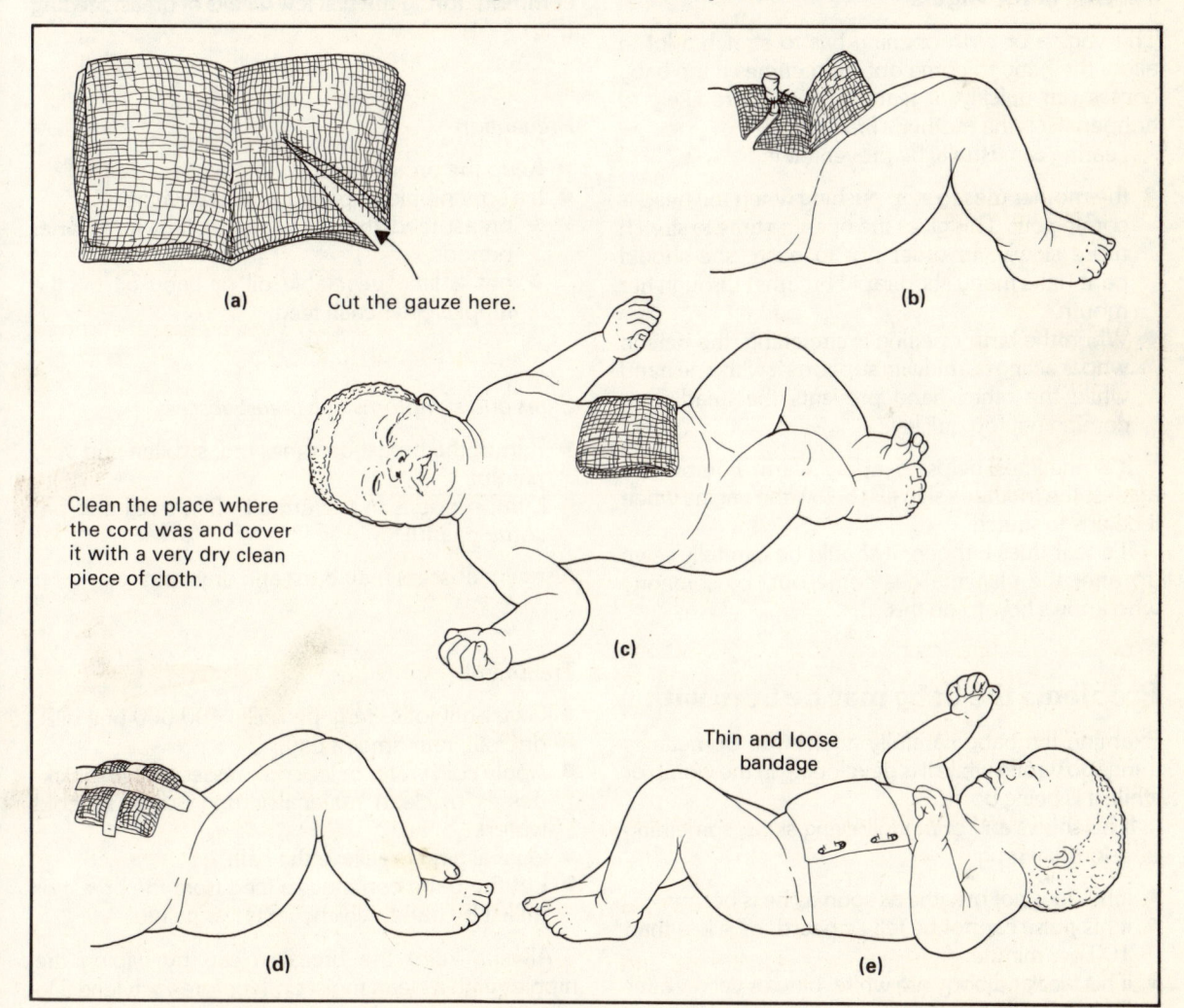

(a) Cut the gauze here.

(b)

(c) Clean the place where the cord was and cover it with a very dry clean piece of cloth.

(d)

(e) Thin and loose bandage

Fig. 9.13 Dressing the cord stump

baby's birth, or if only part of it has appeared, or if the mother is losing more blood, accompany her to a hospital or health centre.

It is normal that the mother should lose about half a litre of blood before and while the afterbirth comes out.

It is not normal that she should lose more blood once the afterbirth is out. If she does, either gently massage the top of her womb or give her an intramuscular injection of oxytocin (the contents of a 5 I.U. ampoule) into her buttock.

If the mother continues to lose blood, give her plenty of liquids to drink and accompany her to a hospital or health centre.

## Tearing of the vagina

The vagina or birth opening has to stretch a lot to allow the baby to come out. Sometimes if the baby comes out quickly, it tears. This is more likely to happen if it is the mother's first baby.

Tearing can usually be prevented if:

- the mother tries to stop pushing when the head is coming out. This gives the opening time to stretch more slowly. In order not to push, she should pant (take many short rapid breaths) through her mouth.
- When the birth opening is stretching, the person who is acting as midwife supports it with one hand while the other hand prevents the head from coming out too quickly.

It sometimes helps to apply warm compresses against the mother's skin just below the vagina when it begins to stretch.

If a tear does happen, it should be carefully sewn up after the placenta has come out, by someone who knows how to do this.

## Problems the baby may be born with

Examine the baby carefully after birth. Sometimes things go wrong while it is developing in the womb or while it is being born.

If he shows any of the following signs, something is seriously wrong:

- if he does not breathe as soon as he is born;
- if his pulse cannot be felt or heard, or is less than 100 per minute;
- if his face and body are white, blue or yellow after he has begun breathing;
- if his arms and legs are floppy or do not move;
- if he grunts or has difficulty in breathing after the first 15 minutes.

Get medical help at once.

If the baby does not pass water or have a bowel movement within 2 days, also get medical advice.

When a woman gives birth after only 7 or 8 months of pregnancy, the baby will be smaller and weaker than a baby born after 9 months pregnancy. Unless this baby is very well looked after he may die, because he is not as strong as a full-term baby.

### Breast abscess

A breast abscess may result from an infection which enters through a sore or cracked nipple. This is most common during the first few weeks of breast feeding (Fig. 9.14).

*Prevention*

- Keep the breast clean.
- If a sore nipple or painful cracks develop:
  - breast-feed the baby more often for shorter periods;
  - put a little vegetable oil or baby oil on the nipples after each feed;

*Signs and symptoms of a breast abscess*

- Part of the breast becomes red, swollen and very painful.
- Lymph nodes in the armpit often swell and become painful.

A severe abscess may burst and drain pus.

*Treatment*

- Give antibiotics (e.g. penicillin 400,000 unit pills, one pill, four times a day);
- Apply cold water or ice compresses (several thicknesses of clean material wrung out in ice-cold water).
- Give aspirin to relieve the pain.
- Let the baby continue to feed from the breast *or* milk it by hand, whichever is less painful.

Always keep the breasts clean by wiping the nipples with a clean moist cloth before each feed. Do not use soap each time as this can also lead to cracking of the skin, sore nipples and infection.

Taking good care of the breasts is important for the health of both the mother and her baby. Breast-feeding should be started on the day of birth. At first the baby may not suck much, but this lets the mother's body get used to his sucking and also prevents sore nipples.

The very first milk the breast makes (called colostrum), although it looks watery, is very good for the baby, as it helps to protect him against infection and contains protein.

One breast hurts a lot

Tell the mother to squeeze the milk from the breast with her hand and to then give this milk to her baby

Apply cold water or ice compresses

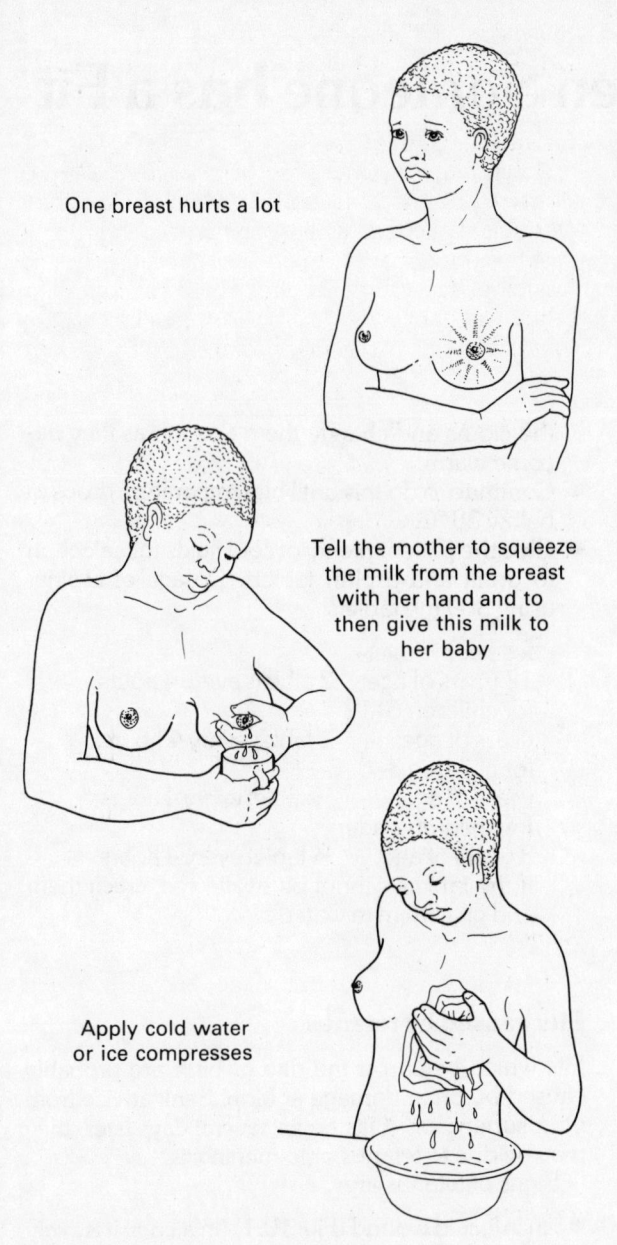

Fig. 9.14 Treating a breast abscess

# 10. What to Do when Someone has a Fit

## Fits

When someone has a fit he makes strange, jerking movements which he cannot control (convulsions) (Fig. 8.10). He may lose consciousness.

In small children, two common causes of fits are a very high fever and severe dehydration (excessive loss of water from the body, probably due to diarrhoea and vomiting). Some babies have small fits when they are cutting their teeth.

Causes also include meningitis, malaria and poisoning. It is a serious sign if a pregnant woman has a fit (see page 52).

Whatever the cause, the immediate treatment is to prevent the patient from hurting himself. Move all furniture, hard, pointed or sharp objects well away from him. Remove any of his clothes which are tight at the waist, neck or across the chest. Also remove anything else which is being worn that may cause injury—e.g. hairpins, artificial teeth, etc.

Keep the patient's airway clear by turning him on his right side. This will also help to prevent him from biting his tongue (Fig. 2.6). Note the pulse, breathing and the time the fit lasts.

If the patient is a pregnant woman, you should get ready for the onset of labour (see page 55). Contact your supervisor for advice if you cannot get the woman to hospital quickly.

### Fits caused by a high fever

A very high fever (over 40 °C) can be dangerous. Your aim will be to bring the patient's temperature down quickly.

*Treatment*
- Strip the patient of all clothes.
- Fan him.
- Either pour tepid (cool, not cold) water over him, or put cloths soaked in tepid water over him. Fan the cloths and change them as soon as they become warm.
- Continue to do this until his temperature drops to below 38 °C.
- Give the patient plenty of cool fluids (not alcohol) to drink and aspirin tablets. Dosage of aspirin: using 300 mg tablets:

  for people over
  12 years of age:     2 tablets every 4 hours;
  for children 6–12
  years of age:        1 tablet every 4 hours;
  for children 3–6
  years of age:        ½ tablet every 4 hours;
  for children under
  3 years of age:      ¼ tablet every 4 hours.

  If the tablets cannot be swallowed, crush them and give them in water.

### Fits caused by tetanus

Fits which begin on the day of birth are probably caused by brain damage at birth. Seek advice from your supervisor. If fits begin several days later, they may be due to tetanus or to meningitis.

Signs of tetanus are:

- an infected wound (Fig. 10.1) (in a baby it is likely to be the cord which is infected; see page 63);
- discomfort or difficulty in swallowing;
- stiff jaw (later muscles of the neck and other parts of the body) (Fig. 10.2);
- painful convulsions (fits): first, painful tightening of the jaw and then the whole body goes into spasms. These fits may be triggered off by moving or touching a person. Sudden noise or light can also bring on the spasms (Fig. 10.3).

In the newborn, the first signs of tetanus usually appear 3–10 days after birth. The baby cries continuously and is unable to suck.

**These wounds are most likely to become dangerously infected:**

dirty wounds, or wounds made with dirty objects

puncture wounds and other deep wounds that do not bleed much

wounds made where animals are kept: in corrals, pig pens etc.

large wounds with severe mashing or bruising

bites, especially from pigs, dogs, or people

bullet wounds

**Wounds very likely to cause tetanus:**

animal bites, especially those of dogs and pigs

gunshot and knife wounds

holes made with dirty needles

puncture wounds from thorns, splinters or nails

injuries caused by barbed wire

**Causes of tetanus in the newborn child:**

the cord has been cut with an instrument that has not been boiled and kept completely clean or

the cord has not been cut **close** to the body or

the newly cut cord is tightly covered or is not kept dry.

when the cord is cut a long way from the body, like this, the chance of tetanus is greater.

Fig. 10.1 *Some of the wounds which are likely to become dangerously infected*

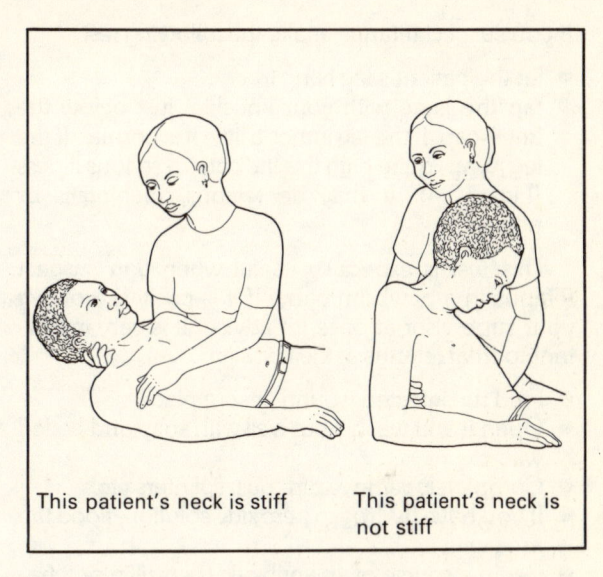

This patient's neck is stiff

This patient's neck is not stiff

Fig. 10.2 *Testing for stiff muscles of the neck*

Sudden noise or bright light may also bring on these spasms

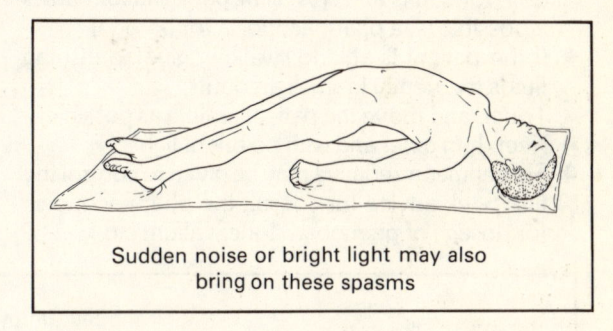

Fig. 10.3 *Spasms caused by tetanus*

*Causes of tetanus in a newborn baby*

Tetanus germs often enter through the umbilical cord of a newborn baby, when there is a lack of cleanliness, and the proper steps to prevent infection are not taken.

The chance of tetanus developing is greater when:

- the cord is cut with an instrument which has not been sterilised (boiled for 5 minutes and kept absolutely clean and covered until used);
- the cord is not cut close to the body (Fig. 10.1);
- the cut cord is tightly covered;
- the cut cord is not kept dry.

Seek medical help at once: tetanus can kill a baby.

64  First Aid

*Treatment*

TESTING FOR TETANUS

If you suspect tetanus, make the following test:

- let the patient's leg hang freely;
- tap the knee with your knuckle, just below the knee-cap. If the leg jumps a little it is normal. If the leg jumps quite high this indicates a serious illness (Fig. 10.4). It may be tetanus, meningitis or poisoning.

This test is especially useful when you suspect tetanus in a newborn baby. If it is positive, contact your supervisor at once for advice. It is very important to treat tetanus at the first sign.

- Find the infected wound or sore place.
- Open it and wash it out well with soap and boiled water.
- Completely remove dirt, pus, splinters etc.
- If you have hydrogen peroxide solution, flood the area with it.
- Begin a course of an antibiotic (penicillin or tetracycline) with a large initial dose (procaine penicillin for adults and crystalline penicillin for babies if possible (see pharmacopoeia for dosage).
- If the patient is able to swallow, give nourishing fluids frequently in small amounts;
- Touch and move the patient as little as possible;
- Keep him quiet and with no bright lights;
- Sometimes a sedative may be given to control the fits. Seek advice (or consult the pharmacopoeia for dosage of phenobarbitone, valium etc.).

Children and adults should be vaccinated against tetanus. This is especially important for pregnant women as their vaccinations protect their new-born babies.

## Fits caused by meningitis

Meningitis is a very serious infection of the brain and is more common in children than in adults. It may begin as a complication of another illness, such as measles, mumps, whooping cough or an ear infection. Children of mothers who have tuberculosis sometimes develop tubercular meningitis during the first year of life.

*Signs and symptoms*

- Fever.
- Severe headache.
- Stiff neck: the child lies with his head and neck bent back (Fig. 10.5).
- Stiff back: the head cannot be put between the legs.
- In babies under 1 year, if the fontanelle (the soft spot at the top of the head) bulges upwards.
- Vomiting.
- Sleepiness.
- Fits (convulsions) or strange jerking movements.
- The child looks very ill and gets worse until he loses consciousness.

If the leg jumps just a little bit, the reaction is normal.

If the leg jumps high, this indicates a serious illness like tetanus (or perhaps meningitis or poisoning with certain medicines or rat poison).

**Test of knee reflexes:** With the leg hanging freely, tap the knee with a knuckle just below the kneecap.

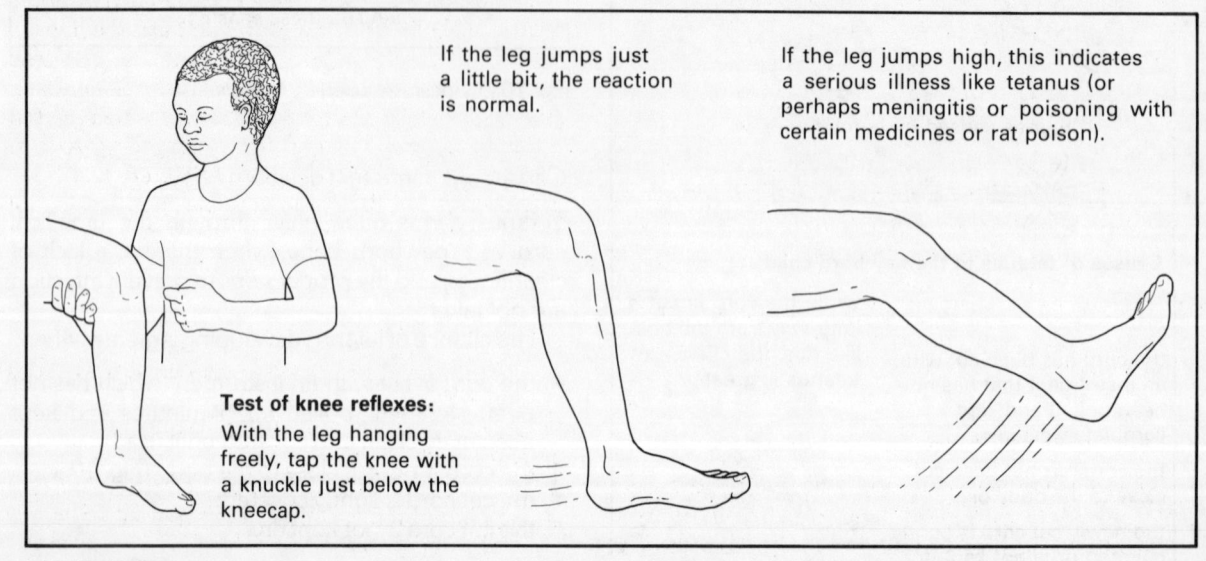

*Fig. 10.4  Testing knee reflexes*

Stiff neck.
The child looks very ill, and lies with his head and neck bent back, like this:

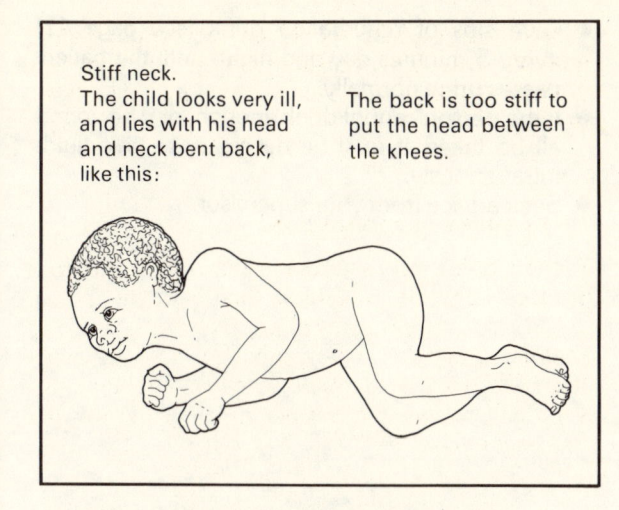

The back is too stiff to put the head between the knees.

*Fig. 10.5 Position of an infant with meningitis*

Tubercular meningitis develops slowly over days or even weeks. Other forms of meningitis come on quickly, developing within days or even hours.

*Treatment*

Obtain medical help quickly: this is a time when every minute is important and the child should have hospital care.
  Meanwhile:

- inject ampicillin or crystalline penicillin (see pharmacopoeia for dosage);
- if the temperature is more than 40 °C, lower it by applying wet cloths and giving aspirin (as described on page 62);
- if you think it is tubercular meningitis, inject the child with streptomycin in addition to the penicillin (see pharmacopoeia for dosage).

Sometimes someone with malaria develops malaria of the brain. As well as the signs and symptoms of malaria, he begins to have fits. Get advice from your supervisor if possible. If not, consult a copy of the pharmacopoeia and inject chloroquine. This should only be given in extreme emergency and you must take great care to see that the dose you give is correct.

## Fits due to epilepsy

Epilepsy causes fits in people who otherwise appear to be fairly healthy. They may occur within hours of each other, or may be days, weeks, months or even years apart.

*Signs and symptoms*

- In some people the fits cause a loss of consciousness.
- The patient may cry out and then fall to the ground.
- His eyes may roll.
- He may froth at the mouth and pass urine.
- He may make violent, jerky movements.
- In mild forms, there may be just momentarily 'blacking-out' incidents, during which the person makes strange sounds and movements or behaves rather strangely for a few seconds.

*Treatment*

- Your main aim is to prevent the patient from harming himself or others (see page 62).
- If the fit lasts a long time, give valium or phenobarbitone (see pharmacopoeia for dosage).
- If the person is sleepy after the fit (even though you have given no sedation), leave him quietly to sleep. In any case, keep the patient quiet until he is fully recovered and feels well again.

The condition is often passed on from one generation to another in families, but it can be controlled by drugs.

## Fits caused by very severe dehydration (lack of water)

Dehydration results when the body loses more liquid than it takes in. The liquid lost can be in the form of vomit, diarrhoea, blood, sweat, etc. It can also happen when a person is too ill to eat or drink. Although people of any age can become dehydrated it develops more quickly and is more dangerous in small children. Any child who has watery diarrhoea is in danger of dehydration if the fluid lost is not replaced quickly.

*Signs and symptoms*

- Little or no urine is passed: what urine is passed is dark yellow.
- Sudden and dramatic loss of weight.
- Dry mouth.
- Sunken eyes, and no tears come with crying.
- Sagging of the fontanelle (soft spot at the top of the head in babies).
- Skin loses its elasticity (stretchiness) (see Fig. 7.1).

In very severe dehydration, these signs and symptoms will be present, but also:

- the pulse will be rapid and weak;
- breathing will be fast and deep; and
- fits may develop.

*Treatment*

- Prevent self-injury during the fits.
- Give sips of rehydration drink (see page 41) every 5 minutes day and night, until the patient passes urine normally.
- If the person cannot drink enough, or if he vomits all he takes, it may be necessary to give fluids intravenously.
- Seek advice from your supervisor.

# 11. What to Do when Someone is Affected by Great Heat or Cold

Under normal circumstances the human body is capable of keeping its own temperature at a level of 36–37 °C. No matter if the weather or the environment is hot or cold, the temperature of the body remains constant. In some circumstances, however, extremes of conditions may upset this balance.

## Heat cramps

In hot weather many people who sweat a lot sometimes get painful cramps in their legs, arms or stomachs because their bodies lack salt (i.e. it has been lost from their bodies in sweat).

*Treatment*

- Give the patient a tumbler of water containing ¼ teaspoonful of salt.
- Add 1 teaspoonful of salt to 1 litre of cool boiled water.
- Tell the patient to drink this mixture three times a day.

The principle behind treatment of cramp is to put the muscles 'on the stretch'.

*Treatment*

- *Foot*: straighten the bent toes by pushing them upwards.
- *Calf*: straighten the knee and bend the foot up at the ankle as far as it will go.
- *Thigh*: straighten the knee and pull the whole leg forward.
- *Hand*: straighten the bent fingers by bending them backwards.

## Heat exhaustion

People who work and sweat a lot may develop heat exhaustion (e.g. people who work in certain manufacturing processes such as mining and steel and iron casting). This may be prevented by taking salt tablets or by drinking large quantities of the mildly salted water as described.

*Signs and symptoms of heat exhaustion*

- Paleness and feeling of weakness.
- Pulse is rapid and weak.
- Cramp pains.

*Treatment*

- Remove the patient to a cool place.
- Raise his feet and rub his legs.
- Give salt tablets or the mildly salted water to drink.

## Heat stroke

Heat stroke is more dangerous (Fig. 11.1). It occurs mainly in older people and in alcoholics during very hot weather.

*Signs and symptoms*

- Fever (sometimes the temperature may be more than 42 °C).
- Red, dry skin.
- The patient may lose consciousness.

*Treatment*

- Place the patient in the shade.
- Soak him with tepid (not cold) water or cover him with cloths wrung out in tepid water (Fig. 11.2).
- Fan, but do not dry him.

68  *First Aid*

**Heat exhaustion**

sweaty, pale, cool skin

large pupils

no fever

weakness

**Heat stroke**

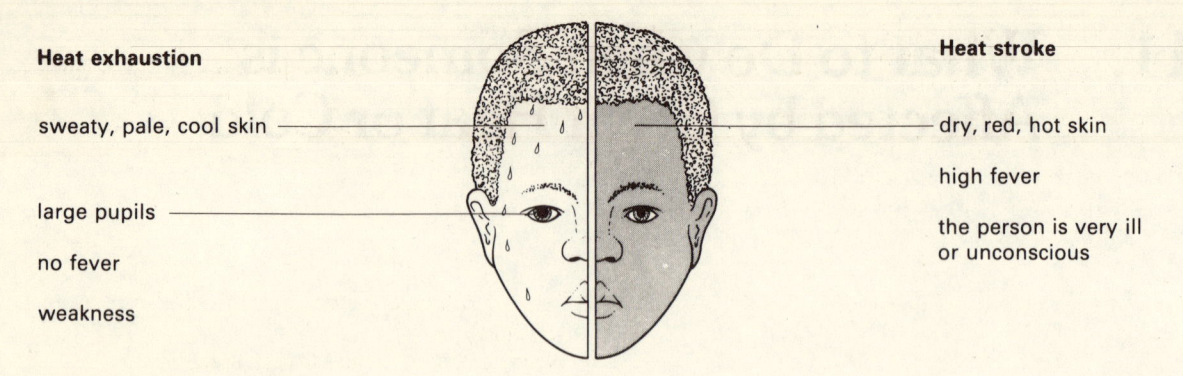

dry, red, hot skin

high fever

the person is very ill or unconscious

*Fig. 11.1 Differences between heat exhaustion and heat stroke*

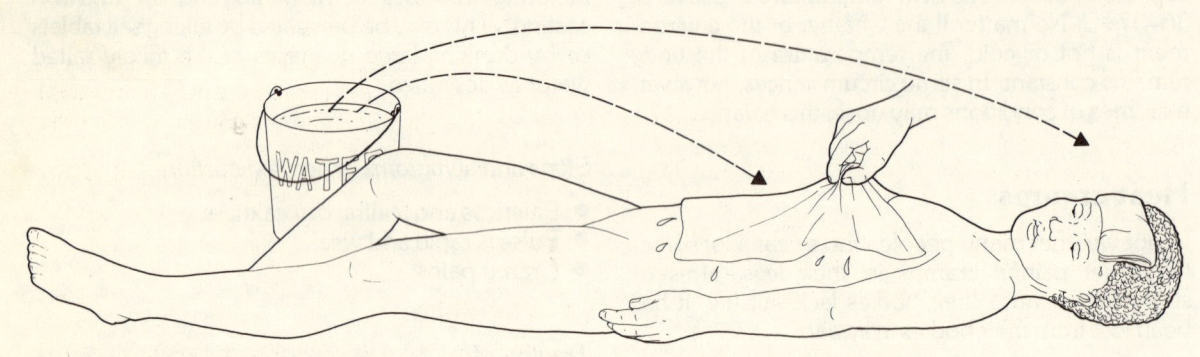

*Fig. 11.2 Reducing the patient's temperature by tepid soaks*

- Repeat the soaking or renew the cloths as soon as they become warm, until the patient's temperature drops.
- Seek advice from your supervisor.
- If there is any burning of the skin, treat as described on page 27.
- If there is pain from the burned area, give aspirin (see pharmacopoeia).

## Hypothermia (temperature below normal)

A fall in the body temperature to below normal may occur in very young babies or in very old people.

### In babies

The newborn baby takes a little time to adjust to the world. In relation to its weight, it also has a larger surface area from which to lose heat. It should therefore be adequately clothed and not left in a draught. If the room in which it is placed is too cold, the baby may develop hypothermia.

*Signs and symptoms*
- Pale.
- Sleepy.
- Reluctant to suck.
- Skin cold to the touch.

*Treatment*
- Warm the baby by wrapping it in a blanket and keeping him in a warm atmosphere.
- If no heat is available, hold the baby carefully wrapped in layers of blankets or an eiderdown.
- Seek advice from your supervisor.

### In very old people

Very old people lose their ability to adjust to cold. Also, because they are old and unsteady, they move slowly and often take little exercise. They therefore make less body heat.

Old people who live alone often do not eat

enough, and so do not make enough heat to keep themselves warm. In addition many cannot afford adequate heating in their homes in cold weather, and therefore may develop hypothermia.

The condition is most often seen in old people who are exposed to cold for a long period, e.g. when they get up at night, slip, break a leg and lie in a cold place for hours until someone finds them.

*Signs and symptoms of hypothermia*

- Sleepiness.
- Confusion.
- Skin pale and cold to touch.
- Weak pulse.

*Treatment*

- Warm the patient by whatever means are available; (e.g. light a fire or stove, close windows and wrap him in blankets or eiderdown). Do not *heat* —just slowly *warm* him.
- Do not warm rapidly: this could do more harm.
- Give hot sweet fluids (help the patient to drink with care if he is confused).
- Seek advice from your supervisor.

## In other people

Hypothermia can also occur in other people if they are exposed to wet, cold conditions and do not take precautions (e.g. when climbing high mountains). The risk is greater if they are injured.

*Signs and symptoms*

- As already described above.
- Rapid mental and physical deterioration, followed by loss of consciousness and death if he is not rescued.

*Treatment*

- Shelter the person from further exposure— wrapping him in a plastic or foil bag to the neck is best, but otherwise whatever is available must be used.
- Carry him to a place of safety.
- Give artificial respiration if required (see page 10).
- Transfer the patient to a warm bed in a warm room.
- Seek guidance from your supervisor.

## Frostbite

Frostbite can occur when the temperature drops below minus 1 °C.

The areas most likely to be frostbitten are the fingers, toes, cheeks, nose and ears.

*Signs and symptoms*

- Intense coldness of the part, followed by loss of sensation.
- When pressed, the tissue feels soft.

*Treatment*

- If the part can be warmed at this stage, recovery can be rapid. The affected part should be covered up, preferably with something woollen, and the person should be wrapped in a rug.
- As soon as possible, the person should be transferred to a warm room.

## Deep frostbite

In a situation where warming cannot take place, and the person remains exposed to severe cold, deep frostbite may occur. In this condition there is a loss of sensation, the area feels very cold to touch, and the tissues when touched are hard.

This condition requires that the patient must be transported to medical attention as quickly as possible.

Once the area has been warmed it must not be allowed to freeze again, and so first aid treatment should **not** be attempted under cold conditions.

If deep frostbite is not treated immediately, fingers, toes, etc. will become gangrenous and will need amputation (cutting off).

## Effects of lightning

During electrical storms, lightning can injure people by striking them. Frequently it strips clothing to shreds, leaving the person exposed.

Shock will be severe and artificial respiration and heart massage may be necessary (see page 14).

Patches of skin may get scorched and will require treatment (see page 27).

If the patient is in contact with metal objects, there may be wounds to treat (see page 18).

# 12. What to Do when Someone Breaks a Bone

A fracture is a break in a bone and is usually the result of violence in one form or another. Fractures caused by direct violence are breaks which occur at the point where they are hit. Indirect violence is said to be the cause when the break occurs some distance from the blow. For example, one or both of the bones of the lower arm (ulnar and radius) are often broken as a result of a fall, when the person puts out an arm to save himself and his weight goes on to the outstretched hand.

Bones can also break as a result of a disease or because of over-use of muscles and tendons (e.g. in people such as athletes).

## Classification (grouping)

Fractures in which there is no break in the skin are described as closed or simple (Fig. 12.1).

When the skin is broken they are called open or compound (Fig. 12.2). (The break in the skin may be the result of injury from the same object as the one which caused the broken bone, and may have occurred at the same time, or it may be caused by the end of a broken bone pushing through muscle and skin.)

When there is damage to other tissues or organs as well, the fracture is called complicated (Fig. 12.3). It is important to bear this possibility in mind when you are treating a patient. For example, fractured ribs can cause lung damage and a fractured skull can cause brain damage. Also, relatively straightforward breaks in the bones of the legs and arms can cause damage to important blood vessels and nerves.

In children the bone sometimes only partly breaks (Fig. 12.4). This is called a greenstick fracture.

*Signs and symptoms of a broken bone*

Signs and symptoms will vary according to where the fracture is and what kind it is.

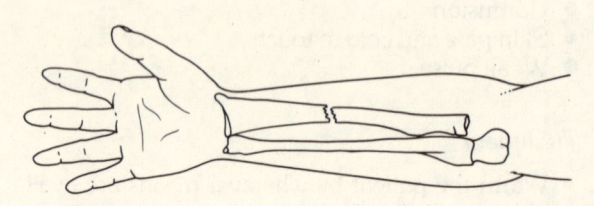

*Fig. 12.1*

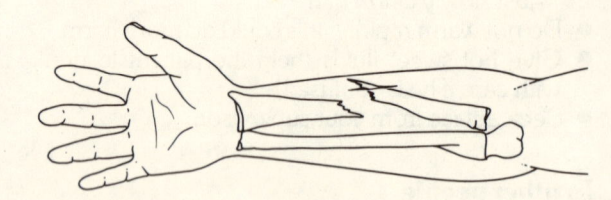

*Fig. 12.2*

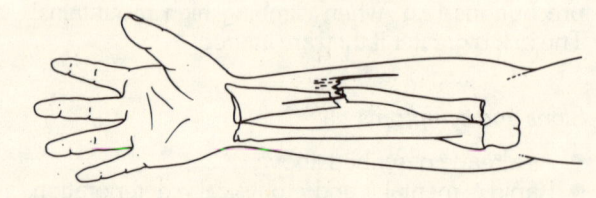

*Fig. 12.3*

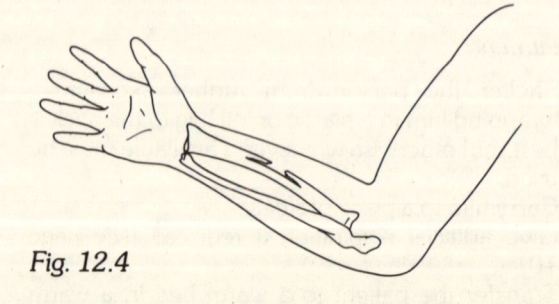

*Fig. 12.4*

*Figs 12.1 to 12.4 Some kinds of fracture*

If you are in any doubt about whether there is a break in a bone, treat the patient as though the bone is broken, until you get advice or help. Ask the patient to keep as still as possible, to prevent making the injury worse.

If there is pain, examine the painful area carefully and gently for swelling and deformity (unusual shape or position). (It helps to decide whether either of these is present if you look at the other side of the body also and compare the two.)

There is always some bleeding around a fracture, even though you may not be able to see it. Sometimes this can be a large amount, and because of this, and the pain, the patient can become shocked. To help prevent this from happening, tell him to lie flat.

*Treatment*

- Treat the patient where he is, unless you are both in danger.
- Move him as little as possible.
- If the fracture is open and there is severe bleeding, this should be dealt with first and a dressing applied. Direct pressure is usually sufficient, although this may be too painful for the patient, in which case, apply pressure to the appropriate pressure point (see page 18).
  Cover the wound (see page 18).
- The broken bone should be immobilised (treated so that it cannot move). This can be done by splinting, including areas above and below the point of the break. You must make quite certain that when splints are used, they are always padded and that they do not interfere with the patient's circulation of blood.
- The patient should then be taken to the health centre or hospital. Keep the broken limb slightly higher than the rest of the patient's body during the journey. This will help to prevent shock and also reduce swelling of the injured part.

## Using splints

All splints should be:

- rigid;
- long enough to go alongside the joint above and below the fracture (Fig. 12.5);
- wide enough to fit the limb comfortably;
- well padded;
- applied, for the journey, over clothing.

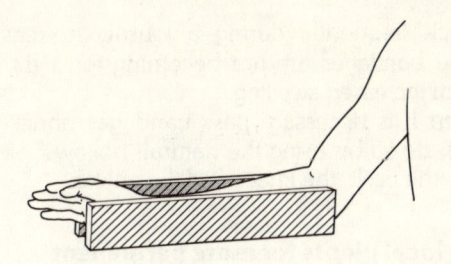

*Fig. 12.5 Extent of splinting*

In emergencies, splints can be improvised by using bamboo, branches of trees, walking sticks, umbrellas, pieces of cardboard and even rolled-up newspapers. Sometimes the patient's own body can be used (e.g. one good leg acting as a splint to the injured one when they are tied together (Fig. 12.6)).

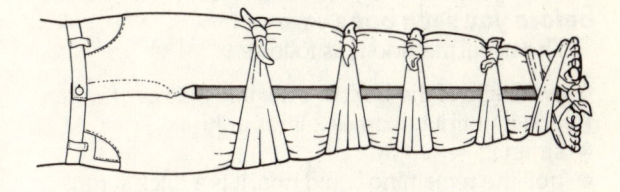

*Fig. 12.6 Splinting by using the patient's own body and figure-of-eight bandage around ankles and feet*

## Bandages

Bandages must be applied firmly to prevent movement but not so tightly that they reduce the circulation of blood or cause pain.

In order to prevent discomfort and soreness of the skin, skin surfaces should be separated with soft padding (i.e. cotton wool or soft cloth) before bandaging.

Always tie knots over the splint or on the uninjured side (Fig. 12.7).

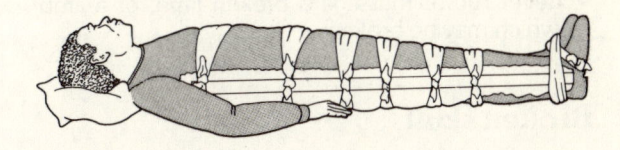

*Fig. 12.7 Splinting for broken femur (upper leg bone) using broad bandaging and tying knots over the splint*

Check frequently during a journey to ensure that the bandages are not becoming too tight because of increased swelling.

When it is necessary pass bandages under the patient, do so by using the natural 'hollows' of the body—the neck, the knees and the ankles.

**Using local plants for more permanent splinting**

If it is not possible to get the patient to medical help for some time, splinting casts can sometimes be made by using the bark of a tree or plant to make a syrup which will dry hard and firm and will not irritate the skin (Fig. 12.8). If you do not know which ones can be used in your area, try out some. Bark from some bean trees is often good, and the stem and sap from many of the tree-climbing plants can also be used (e.g. arum lily).

**Always contact your supervisor for advice before you set a bone yourself.**

The usual method is as follows:

- put a kilo of the bark or stalk into 5 litres of water;
- boil it until it becomes 2 litres only;
- strain it;
- boil the remaining liquid until it is a thick syrup;
- dip strips of flannel or other clean cloth in the syrup and use as follows:
  - make sure the bone is in a good, normal position;
  - wrap the arm or leg in soft dry cloth (**never** put a cast directly on to the skin and **never** put one on over a cut or open wound);
  - apply a layer of cotton or kapok;
  - wrap the wet syrupy strips so that they form a cast which is firm but not too tight (Fig. 12.9). Even if the cast is not tight when you put it on, the limb may swell later and make it too tight. If this happens, or if the fingers or toes are cold or blue, take off the cast at once and put on another looser one.
  - look at the fingers or toes frequently yourself, and tell the patient to let you know if they become uncomfortable, blue or cold.
- never rub or massage a broken limb, or a limb which may be broken.

## Broken skull

Fractures of the skull are not necessarily important. They become so when the bone is depressed (dented), causing damage to the brain underneath

Make sure the bones are in a good position

Do **not** put the cast directly against the skin.

Wrap the arm or leg in a soft cloth.

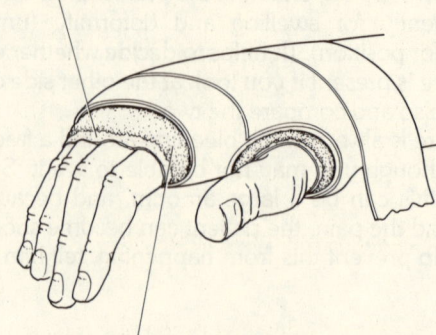

Then follow with a layer of cotton or wild kapok.

Finally, put on the wet cloth strips so that they form a cast that is firm but not too tight.

It is important that the cast covers enough of the arm or leg to keep the broken bones from moving – usually the joint above and the joint below the break.

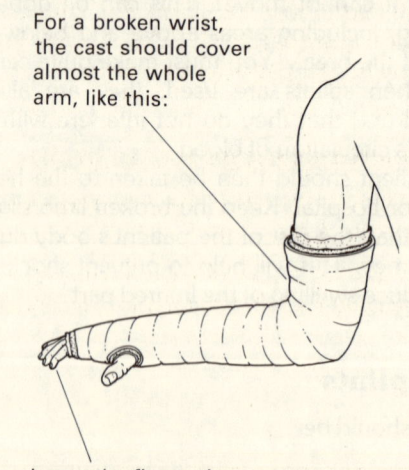

For a broken wrist, the cast should cover almost the whole arm, like this:

Leave the finger tips uncovered so that you can see if they keep a good colour.

*Fig. 12.8 Using local plants for making a cast*

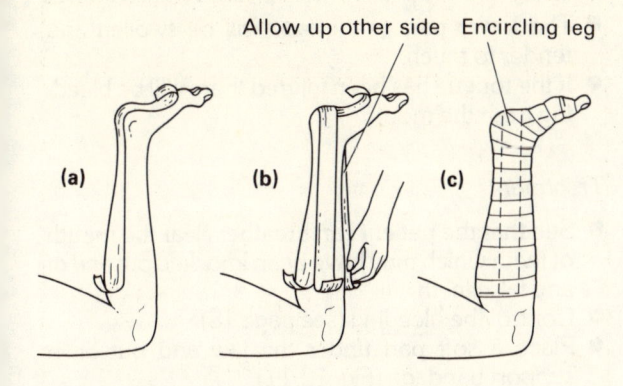

*Fig. 12.9 Applying a cast to a broken limb*

it, or when there is damage to the blood vessels and there is bleeding.

An uncomplicated fractured skull requires no treatment and will heal naturally. The patient may, however, require treatment for cuts (see page 18) or for concussion (stunning) (see page 31).

## Fractures of the base of the skull

These are difficult to diagnose.

*Signs and symptoms*

- There may be blood loss from the ear and nose (sometimes this is swallowed and later vomited).
- Colourless fluid from the spine may also come from the ear and nose.
- There may be bruising around the eyes.

## Patients with damage to the brain

The two main points to remember when caring for a patient with brain damage are:

- make certain that his breathing is adequate;
- avoid any action which could make his condition worse.

*Treatment*

- If the brain is visible outside the wound, it should **not** be cleaned and **no pressure** should be applied. A light, clean, preferably sterile (if you have it) dressing, such as a piece of sterile gauze, should be held in place by a loose bandage (Fig. 12.10).

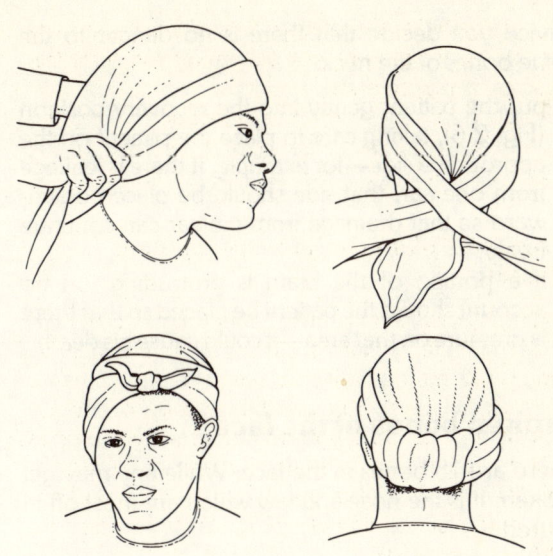

*Fig. 12.10 Dressing an open head wound with a loose head bandage*

- If it is possible to raise slightly the top part of the patient's body, this should be done, but the head should **not** be placed on a pillow or on rolled-up cloth, as this could cause further damage to the spinal cord and/or block the airway.
- Even if the patient appears to be bright and alert when you arrive on the scene, you should continue to observe him carefully because worsening can be very sudden. You should be prepared to undertake artificial respiration and/or cardiac massage at any time.
- A particularly close watch should be kept on the patient's pupils (see page 4). A dilated (large) pupil reacting (responding) slowly to light is a sign of increasing pressure from blood on that side of the brain. A slow pulse rate also means raised pressure within the skull.
- Seek advice from your supervisor and arrange for transport to hospital.

Sometimes abnormal electrical activity in the brain follows injury, and this could result in the patient having a fit. You should remember that stoppage of breathing during such an attack may not mean a blocked airway. It is usually due to spasms of the muscles.

On no account put your fingers into the patient's mouth while he is having a fit.

If, after very careful examination, thought and

74     First Aid

advice you decide that there is no danger to the spine bones of the neck:

- put the patient gently into the recovery position (Fig. 2.6), taking care to place the patient on the appropriate side—for example, if there is leakage from one ear, that side should be placed downward so that drainage from the ear can continue freely;
- if a portion of the brain is protruding, on no account should the patient be placed so that there is pressure on that area—it could cause his death.

## Broken bones of the face

There are 18 bones in the face. While any may get broken, it is the nose and jaw which are most often injured.

*Signs and symptoms*

- Bleeding, probably from the nose and mouth.
- Severe swelling (which could block the airway).

*Treatment*

Cuts on the face often bleed briskly, but you should not let your attention be focused on them. They are rarely serious and other conditions or injuries should be dealt with first.

On arrival, check for:

- signs of obstruction to the airway (see page 4);
- serious bleeding which could threaten life (see page 2);
- the level of consciousness (see page 4).

You should remember that if the damage is sufficient to render the patient unconscious, there may be brain and/or spinal cord damage. Handle him very carefully indeed (see page 75).

Get information on what happened from people standing by (see page 1).

## Fractured jaw

*Signs and symptoms of a broken jaw bone (usually only one side of the jaw is broken)*

- There may be pain, especially when the jaw is moved (when talking or swallowing).
- There may be a lot of saliva mixed with blood.
- Teeth may have been knocked out or loosened.

- The lower part of the face will be swollen and tender to touch.
- If the tongue has been injured there will be bleeding from the mouth.

*Treatment*

- See that the patient can breathe: clear the mouth of teeth which may have been knocked out and of any false teeth.
- Control the bleeding (see page 18).
- Place a soft pad under the jaw and put on a support bandage (Fig. 12.11).
- If the patient is unconscious, place him in the recovery position (see Fig. 2.6), keeping the jaw well forward (see Fig. 2.3).
- Remove the patient to hospital as soon as possible.

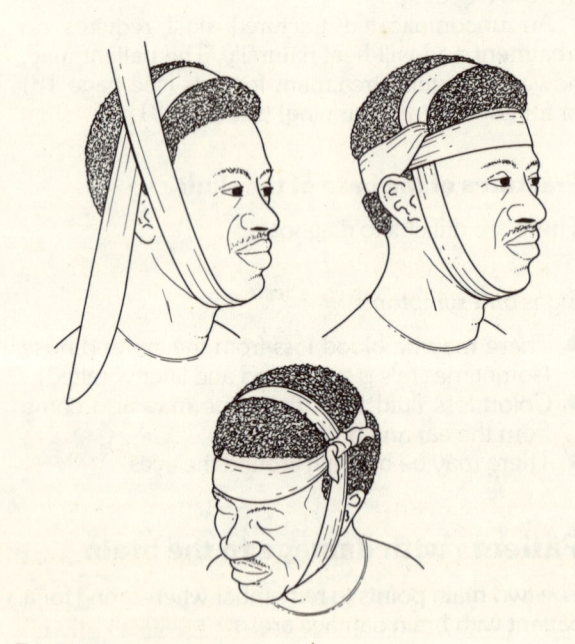

*Fig. 12.11  Jaw bandage*

## Injury to the spine

Fracture of the spine (broken back) calls for the utmost care. The spinal cord can be permanently damaged by rough or incorrect handling, and this leads to life-long disability or even to death.

Fracture of the spine should always be suspected in all instances where there is a history of accidental injury to the back and there is pain. It may, however, be made more difficult by injury to the spinal cord which runs inside the bones of the spine (Fig. 12.12). When this has happened there is either complete or partial loss of power or sensation (feeling) or both, below the waist or the place where the injury is. This can be due to:

- a fall from a height on to the back, or on to a wall or bar;
- a fall of a heavy weight across the patient's back;
- a fall on to the head (especially in diving);
- a heavy fall on to the feet or buttocks;
- over-stretching of the spine in a motor-car crash.

If the patient is unconscious, the fact that he has a spinal injury may not cross your mind.

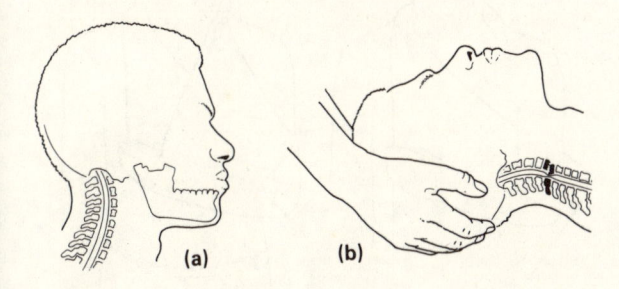

*Fig. 12.12 (a) spinal cord—normal position and (b) spinal cord injury—displaced vertebra*

*Signs*

- Bruising, grazing or other injury to the face or forehead.
- Unusual dryness of the skin of the lower part of the body.
- Complete limpness and lack of movement of two or all four limbs.
- No reaction to movement of obviously injured limbs.
- A see-saw movement of the body during breathing.

**Any movement, especially of the neck, must be carried out with the greatest care possible.**

*Treatment*

- Even when there is no apparent loss of movement or feeling, handle the patient with very great care.
- Warn him to remain still.
- If you are not in a dangerous place, do not move the patient until you have skilled help.
- Take measures to prevent shock (see pages 6-7).
- If the patient is conscious you should ask him about numbness, weakness and any inability to move any part of his body, as well as about pain and other injuries (but do not ask him **to** move: only whether he **can**).
- If he is unable to move his limbs, they should be examined very carefully for injury, but **very, very** carefully because there will be no pain to warn the patient or you about other fractures and wounds. Swelling and deformity should also be looked for.
- Treat any other injuries you find.
- If the patient is able to move his back without pain or difficulty, he is unlikely to have a fractured spine. It is emphasised that he should only be asked if he **can** move. He should **not** be instructed to move and must **never** be made to move.
- Get the patient to medical help as soon as possible.

## Preparation for transport to hospital

The general rule for handling a patient with any broken bone is that he must be prevented, as far as possible, from causing the bone or bones to move. This is most important when bones of the spine are broken. If the patient is unconscious, even greater care must be taken because he will not be able to tell you when movement is painful.

While distorted arms and legs may be straightened gently, a distorted spine must **never** be. The patient's original position (that in which he was found), should be supported by pads, pillows, etc. Sandbags or tightly rolled clothing should be placed either side of his head to stop it from moving.

If the patient's position has to be moved because of other dangers (e.g. fire), it must be done with the spine being held 'all in one piece'—with the head, shoulders and hips in the same position. To do this you will need several people and someone experienced and skilled to coordinate their movements (see page 88).

Even if it is only a short journey to hospital, you **must** take precautions to avoid pressure on the skin which has no feeling in it—sores from pressure can develop within an hour of injury. Therefore:

- place the patient on a firm, smooth surface which supports him well;
- smooth any wrinkled or crumpled clothing underneath him;

- remove any hard objects (such as keys, and money in a back trouser pocket) from underneath him;
- fill in the natural hollows of the body (neck, knees and ankles) very gently with small pads of soft cloth, making certain you do not change his position;
- support his head with other small pads;
- protect his bony prominences—ankles, wrists and so on, from pressure;
- place pads under his calves, if he is on his back, or between his knees and feet if he is lying on his side;
- place pads very gently under his hips;
- loosen any tight constrictions, such as straps, braces, shoes, laces and belts.

If several hours pass before you arrive at a hospital, the patient's position should be changed every 2 hours to prevent pressure sores from forming. Make certain your helpers know what they are doing, why they are doing it, and how to do it well and all together. One person should take the patient's legs, the second person should take his shoulders and hips, and the third should take his head and neck. **All must turn the patient together, keeping his position unaltered**.

Readjust all pads each time.

If the patient also has a broken leg or legs, it is better not to splint. If you do use splints (because the journey is going to be long and on uneven ground), pad them very well. Protect both legs—even if one is not injured—from any pressure which may be caused by splints and knots in bandages.

## Broken breast bone (sternum)

This kind of injury is usually the result of crushing. Underlying organs (e.g. lungs) may also be injured.

*Treatment*

- Loosen any tight clothing around the neck, chest or waist.
- Place the patient in the semi-recumbent position (Fig. 2.18) if this is comfortable for him.
- Seek advice from your supervisor if you think organs are also damaged.
- Transport to hospital.

## Broken collar bone (clavicle)

A fractured collar bone is usually caused by falling on to an outstretched hand.

*Signs and symptoms*

- The patient will probably hold the arm on the injured side, with his other hand.
- His head may be inclined towards the injured side to help relieve the pain by lessening the pull of the muscles.
- There may be swelling and deformity at the actual place where the break is.

*Treatment*

- Brace the shoulders.
- Place the arm in a sling (Fig. 12.13).

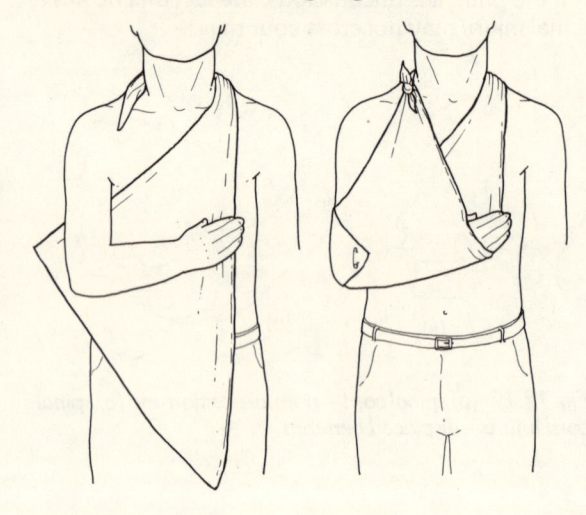

*Fig. 12.13 Arm sling*

## Broken bone of the upper arm (humerus)

*Signs and symptoms*

- Pain.
- Swelling.
- Deformity (usually).

*Treatment*

A broken upper arm is best treated by:

- using the upper part of the patient's body as a splint.

If the elbow is not broken:

- the arm should be gently bent and a sling applied (Fig. 12.14);

- it should then be secured to the patient's body, using two bandages, scarves, ties, belts or strips of cloth; one below the break and one above it.

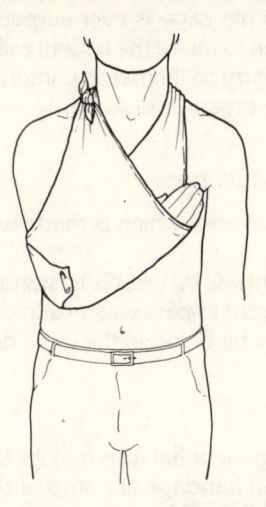

*Fig. 12.14 Treatment of a broken arm when the elbow is not broken*

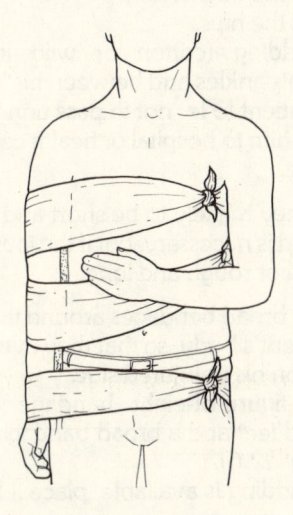

*Fig. 12.15 Treatment of a broken arm when the elbow is also injured*

If the elbow cannot be bent:
- do not force bending;
- lay the patient down;
- gently position the arm to his side, his palm against his thigh;
- place soft padding between his arm and body;

- bandage with three broad bandages—tie them on the patient's uninjured side:
  - round his upper arm and body,
  - round the forearm and body, and
  - round the wrist and thighs (Fig. 12.15);
- transport by stretcher to health centre or hospital.

## Broken bones of the lower arm (radius and ulnar)

- If a break in either the radius, ulnar or both is suspected, the arm should be supported in a sling.
- A plaster cast may be applied if the break is simple and the bone does not need to be put back into its proper place. The cast should go up to the fingers and finish just below the elbow.
- Take all necessary care to ensure that it is not too tight (see page 72).

## Broken fingers (carpals and metacarpals)

- Broken fingers should be strapped to uninjured ones.
- Put the arm in a sling.
- Broken fingers may also be cut, and you will need to treat the bleeding part of the hand as well (see page 22). Remember that if you have no suitable material for making an arm sling, you should pin the patient's sleeve of the injured arm to the front of his coat on the other side.

## Broken ribs

Ribs may be broken by either direct or indirect force.

If the force has been direct there may be a complicated fracture with damage to the lungs.

When there has been indirect force, more than one rib will probably be broken because of pressure on both the back and the front of the chest.

*Signs and symptoms*

- Breathing will be shallow and rapid (this is because of the body's effort to lessen pain by limiting movement).
- If there is damage to the lungs there will be the signs and symptoms given on page 9.

## First Aid

*Treatment*

If the lungs are not injured:

- put the arm on the injured side into a sling.

If the lungs are injured:

- make any 'sucking' wound airtight (see page 21);
- put the arm on the injured side into a sling;
- lay the patient down in the semi-recumbent position, and turned on to his injured side (Fig. 12.16);
- prop him in this position by putting clothes or blankets folded lengthways along his back;
- remove the patient on a stretcher to hospital as soon as possible.

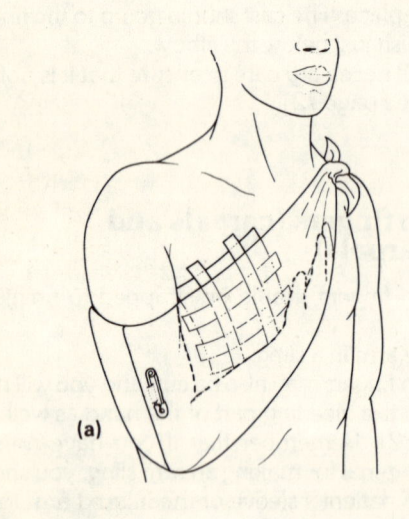

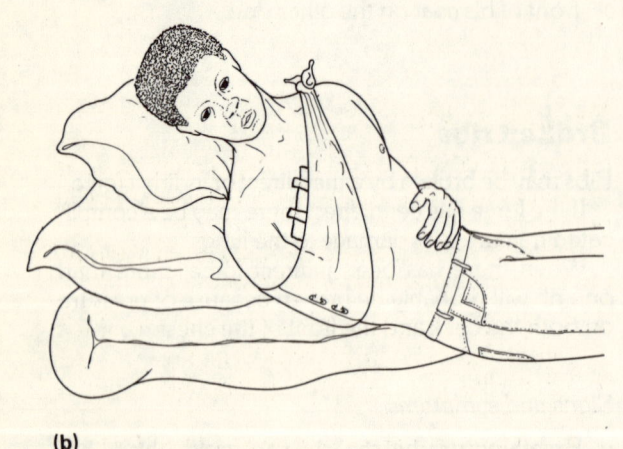

*Fig. 12.16 Treatment for broken ribs (a) first stage and (b) second stage*

## Broken hip cage (pelvis)

The pelvis is the bony basin enclosing the lower part of the body and sometimes called the hip cage. If a break in this hip cage is ever suspected, great care must be taken to move the patient as little as possible to prevent injury to the pelvic contents (the bladder, reproductive organs and so on).

*Signs and symptoms*

- Pain in that area which is made worse by movement.
- The patient will be unable to stand.
- He may want to pass water (urine) frequently.
- There may be blood in the urine he passes.

*Treatment*

- Place the patient flat with his legs together.
- Tie a broad bandage or a strip of cloth:
  - around the ankles;
  - around the knees;
  - around the thighs; and
  - around the hips.
- Place padding (cotton or wild kapok, etc.) between his ankles and between his knees.
- Tell the patient to try not to pass urine.
- Transport him to hospital or health centre as soon as possible.

If the journey is likely to be short and smooth, no further first aid is necessary, but if the journey is likely to be delayed or rough and long:

- Apply two broad bandages around the lower part of the patient's body, so that they overlap by half. Tie them on his uninjured side.
- Apply a figure-of-eight bandage around his ankles and feet and a broad bandage around his knees (Fig. 12.6).
- If more padding is available, place it between his thighs.

## Fractured shoulder blade (scapula)

It is not very often that a shoulder blade is broken. When it is, it is usually as a result of direct force or violence.

*Signs and symptoms*

- Pain.
- Swelling.

*Treatment*

- Remove the patient's coat.
- Place a pad in his armpit on the affected side.
- Place his arm in a sling with his fingertips pointing to the opposite shoulder.
- Secure the arm to his chest by tying a broad bandage over the sling.
- Transport him to hospital or health centre.

## Broken leg bones (femur or tibia and fibula)

*Signs and symptoms*

- Pain.
- Swelling.
- Deformity.

The injured leg is likely to be shorter than the other and the foot on that side will be twisted outwards. (If the ends of the bone are forced against each other (impacted fracture), this does not happen.)

If an old person falls, and says that he has pain in the hip, he should be considered to have broken the neck of the thigh bone (femur).

*Treatment*

For all broken legs:

- hold and keep the injured leg still;
- bring the leg which is not injured gently to the side of the injured one, and tie both legs together;
- send the patient to hospital.

If the journey is long, do the following:

(a) WHEN BONES OF THE LEG BELOW THE KNEE ARE BROKEN

- Apply a well-padded splint between the legs from the top of the patient's thigh to his foot.
- Secure this by tying together with broad bandages:
  - the ankles and feet (with a figure-of-eight bandage);
  - the knees;
  - the legs;
  - the thighs;
  - below the break (see Fig. 12.7).
- Arrange for the casualty to be taken to hospital.

(b) WHEN THE BONE ABOVE THE KNEE IS BROKEN

- Apply a well-padded splint between the legs and an additional long padded splint to the affected side, extending from the armpit to the foot;
- Apply seven bandages:
  - five as previously described above, one around the chest (just below the armpits), and one around the hips.

## Broken knee-cap (patella)

A broken knee-cap may be the result of direct force or muscular action (e.g. playing football).

- Splint the leg from ankle to thigh.
- Place soft padding under the patient's ankle to raise his heel off the splint (Fig. 12.17).
- Raise his leg slightly to prevent swelling.
- Send to hospital or a health centre.

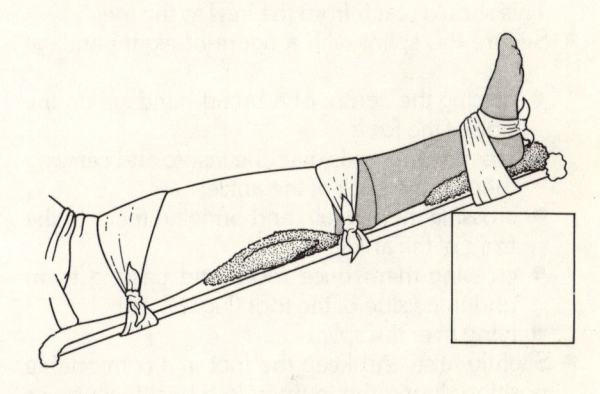

*Fig. 12.17 Treatment for broken knee cap*

## Broken ankle

Often it is difficult to know whether an ankle is broken or sprained, and an X-ray is the only way to be certain.

If there is any doubt and an X-ray is not possible, the ankle should be treated as broken.

- Apply an L-shaped splint along the side of the patient's foot and up the back of his leg.
- Secure the splint by applying three bandages as follows:
  - a figure-of-eight around his ankle and foot;
  - a broad bandage around his thigh;
  - a broad bandage around his lower leg.
- Transport the patient to hospital or health centre, with the injured limb slightly raised.

## Broken foot bones (tarsals and metatarsals)

A foot is usually injured by crushing—a heavy weight dropping on, or passing over, it. e.g. a motor-car.

*Signs and symptoms*

- Pain.
- Swelling.
- Loss of movement.

*Treatment*

- Remove shoe or boot and sock or stocking.
- Treat any wound.
- Apply a well-padded splint to the side of the foot. This should reach from the heel to the toes.
- Secure this splint with a figure-of-eight bandage by:
  - placing the centre of a broad bandage on the side of the foot;
  - crossing the ends over the instep and carrying them to the back of the ankle;
  - crossing them again and bringing them to the front of the ankle;
  - crossing them once more and passing them under the side of the foot (Fig. 12.18);
  - tying over the splint.
- Slightly raise and keep the foot in a comfortable position during the journey to a health centre or hospital.

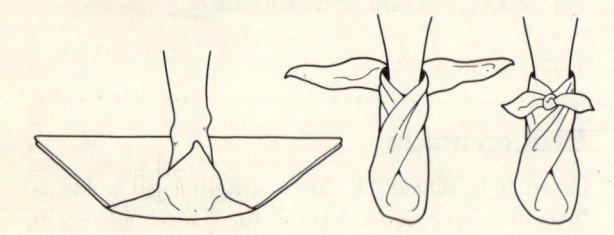

*Fig. 12.18 Bandage for broken feet*

## For all fractures

- Give pain-killers if necessary and if the patient's condition allows this.
- Transport to hospital or health centre carefully, quickly and gently (chapter 14).
- If it is not possible to transfer the patient to hospital or health centre for a plaster cast, you may be able to make one yourself (see page 72).

- **It is very important to see that the bone is in a good position before you apply a cast. Permanent deformity can result if a bone is badly set.**

## Sprains

Sometimes it is difficult to know whether a joint, especially an ankle, is broken or sprained; but if the patient can walk, he is unlikely to have a fracture.

A sprain is a tearing of either ligaments (short bands binding bones together), muscles or the covering of joints (capsules).

*Signs and symptoms*

- Pain especially on movement.
- Swelling.
- Colouring (bruising) of the area some hours later.

*Treatment*

- Raise the limb.
- Put a cold compress (several thicknesses of material wrung out in iced water), over the area.
- Renew the compresses when they get warm and dry.
- Bandage firmly with a crêpe bandage (Fig. 12.19).

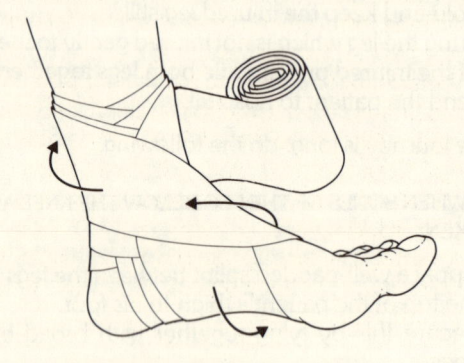

*Fig. 12.19 Bandage for a sprained ankle*

## Strains

A strain occurs when a muscle is over-stretched or gets tired.

There is no tearing and no swelling.

The treatment is the same as that given for a sprain.

Rest should be continued until there is no pain.

# 13. What to Do when Something is Wrong with the Eye, the Ear, the Nose, or the Mouth

## The eye

Eyes are extremely delicate, and good care should be taken of them. When an eye is injured, treatment should be given immediately. Some injuries or conditions are serious, and for these medical help should be obtained as quickly as possible. These are:

(a) a wound which cuts or pierces the eyeball;
(b) a blow which causes the eye to fill with blood (Fig. 13.1);
(c) great pain inside the eye (the diagnosis is probably iritis or glaucoma) (Fig 13.2);
(d) a difference between the sizes of the pupils (Fig. 13.3) (the diagnosis is probably brain damage, poisoning, stroke, injury to the eye, or glaucoma or iritis, but remember that some difference is normal in a few people);
(e) the sight begins to fail in one eye or in both;
(f) a painful greyish spot on the clear (transparent) layer which covers the iris and the pupil of the eye (the cornea) with redness around the cornea (the diagnosis is probably corneal ulcer) (Fig. 13.4);
(g) an infection or inflammation of an eye which does not get better after 5 days of treatment with an antibiotic ointment.

This starts suddenly with a headache or severe pain in the eye. The eye becomes red, the vision blurred. The eyeball feels hard to the touch, like a marble. There may be vomiting. The pupil of the bad eye is bigger than that of the good eye.

Normal

Glaucoma

If not treated very soon, acute glaucoma will cause blindness within a few days. Surgery is often needed. **Get medical help quickly.**

*Fig. 13.2 Acute glaucoma*

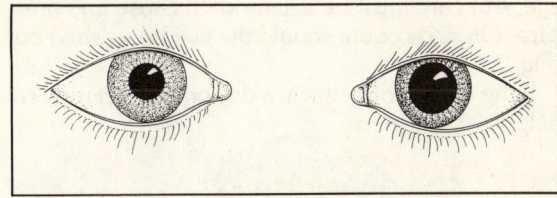

*Fig. 13.3 Difference in the size of pupils*

Corneal ulcer     Corneal scar

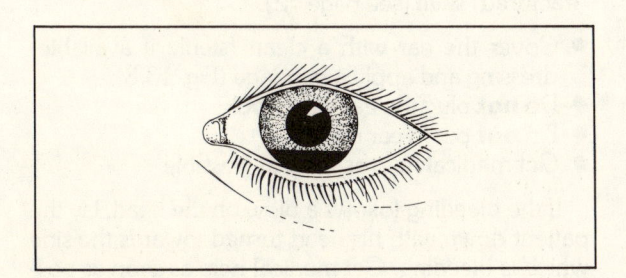

*Fig. 13.1 Bleeding behind the cornea*

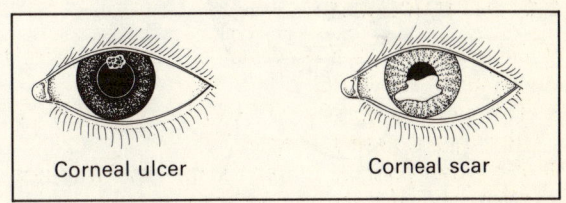

*Fig. 13.4 Corneal ulcer and scar*

## Injuries to the eye

All injuries to the eyeball are serious, for they may result in blindness. Even small cuts of the cornea, if not treated correctly, may become infected and affect the sight in that eye. It is especially dangerous if the black area under the white layer of the eye is injured; also when the eye becomes filled with blood after it has been hit, e.g. by a fist in a fight. Medical help should be sought as soon as possible. (*NB*: A painless blood-red patch in the white of the eye sometimes appears after coughing hard or lifting something heavy (Fig. 13.5). This is the result of a burst small blood vessel. It is harmless and will disappear slowly without being treated.)

Foreign bodies entering the eye at speed, e.g. pieces of glass following a windscreen accident, may perforate the cornea and remain inside the eye. The condition is painful and serious, and the victim requires hospital treatment. Meanwhile he will probably close his injured eye because of the pain and there is nothing that the first-aider can do except comfort him during the journey.

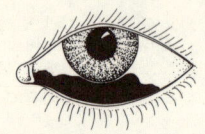

*Fig. 13.5 Bleeding in the white of the eye*

## Treatment for eye injuries

A **very light** covering may be applied to an injured eye, but care must be taken not to cause any pressure. On no account should the eye be washed out (Fig. 13.6).

If the eye is not better in a day or two, get medical help.

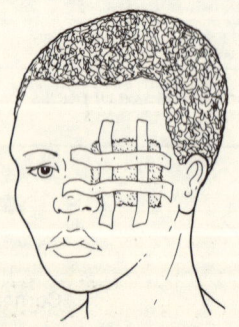

*Fig. 13.6 Light eye dressing*

## Foreign bodies in the eye

A foreign body can be a speck of dust or ash, particle of sand, or a small fly, etc.

Often you can get a piece of dirt or sand out of the eye by flooding it with tepid boiled water. If this does not work:

- instruct the patient not to rub his eye;
- while the patient looks up, gently draw the lower lid down and out;
- if the foreign body is seen on the lower lid, remove it with a moistened wisp of cotton wool or the corner of a clean handkerchief;
- if the particle is thought to be under the upper lid, then, while the patient looks down, grasp the upper lid and draw it down and out over the lower lid. This should wipe away the foreign body.

If it does not:

- stand behind the patient;
- carefully place a smooth matchstick at the base of the upper lid and press it gently backwards;
- while the patient looks down, grasp the lashes of the upper lid and pull and turn it inside out over the matchstick (Fig. 13.7);
- remove foreign body with a wisp of cotton wool or the moistened tip of a handkerchief corner.

Do not try to remove a foreign body from the eyeball. Refer the patient to the health centre or hospital.

If an acid or alkali (e.g. caustic soda) gets into the eyes, this can be very dangerous. Flood the eyes with running water for several minutes. Get medical advice as soon as possible.

## The ear

### Bleeding from the ear

Bleeding from the ear may be due to a broken (fractured) skull (see page 72).

- Cover the ear with a clean (sterile if available) dressing and apply a bandage (Fig. 13.8).
- Do **not** plug the ear with wool.
- Do **not** put in ear drops.
- Get medical help as soon as possible.

If the bleeding follows a blow on the head, lay the patient down with his head turned towards the side which is bleeding. Get medical help as soon as possible.

*Eyes, Ears, Nose, and Mouth* 83

Hold the edge of the eyelid between the thumb and the index finger. Gently pull it down a little.

Fold the eyelid back onto a match held in the other hand.

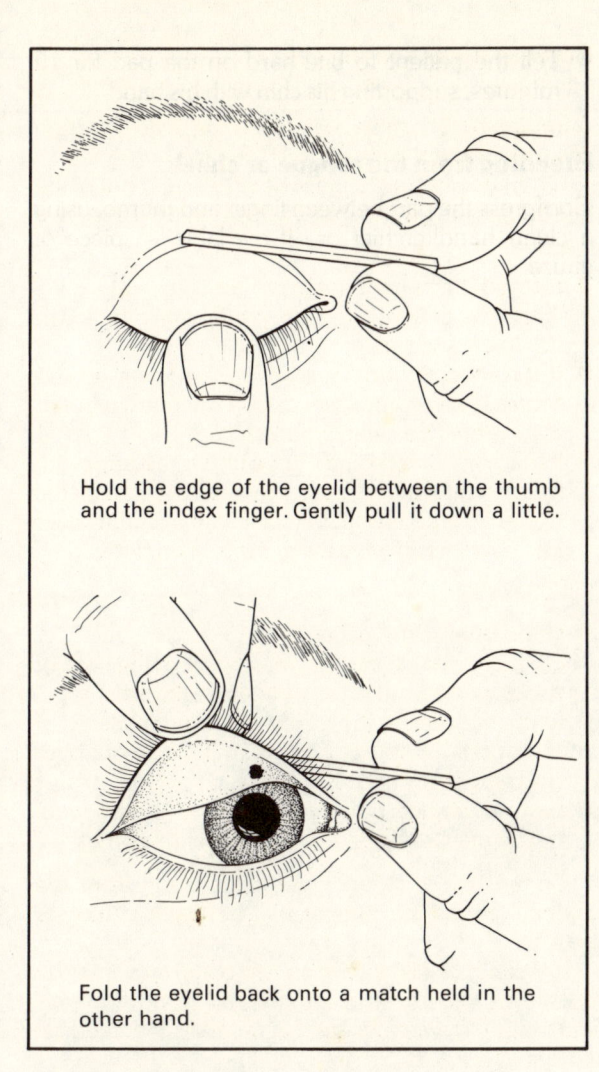

*Fig. 13.7 How to fold the eyelid back to remove something from the eye*

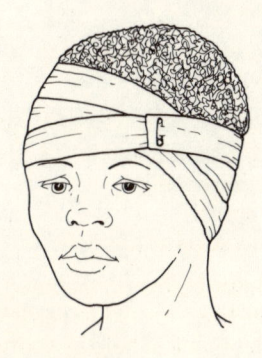

*Fig. 13.8 Ear bandage*

## Foreign body in the ear

Turn the patient's head to the side: the foreign body may drop out.

If it is an insect which is inside the ear, lay the patient down with that ear uppermost. Direct a torch-light to the ear—the insect may follow the light and come out of the ear. If this does not succeed:

- pour in tepid boiled water: the insect may float out.

If neither of these treatments is successful, seek medical help.

## The nose

### Bleeding from the nose

- Get the patient to pinch the lower part of his nose firmly for 10 minutes, while breathing through his mouth (Fig. 13.9).
- Loosen tight clothing around his neck.
- Tell the patient not to blow his nose for several hours.
- If bleeding persists, obtain medical advice.

If bleeding from the nose follows a blow or injury to the head it may be due to a fractured skull (see page 72).

1. Sit quietly

2. Pinch the nose firmly for 10 minutes or until the bleeding has stopped.

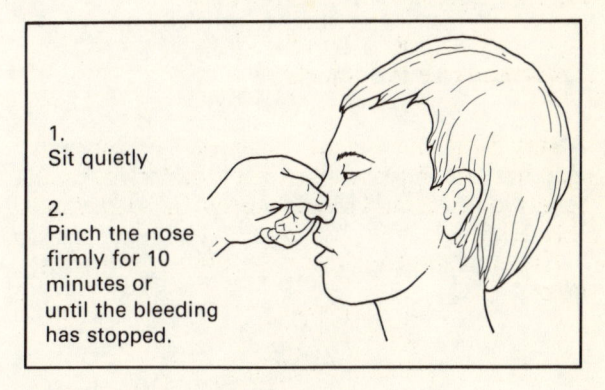

*Fig. 13.9 How to stop a nose bleed*

### Foreign body in the nose

In an adult, a foreign body may enter the nose by accident, but most commonly the patient is a child who has inserted a pea or a bean into his nose.

Do not attempt to remove it. Get medical help.

## The mouth

### Bleeding from a tooth socket

- Sit the patient down.
- Put a small pad of lint or gauze over, but not deeply in the socket. This should be large enough to keep upper and lower teeth apart when bitten on.
- Tell the patient to bite hard on the pad for 15 minutes, supporting his chin with his hand.

### Bleeding from the tongue or cheek.

Compress the part between finger and thumb, using a clean handkerchief or—if available—a piece of gauze.

# 14. How to Take a Patient to Medical Help

There are many methods of carrying patients to help: all need to be practised under supervision.

Your aim is to see that the patient reaches his destination without his condition becoming worse. The following principles must always be kept in mind:
(1) The position in which the patient has put himself, or in which he has been placed, must not be altered unless there is a very good reason.
(2) Throughout transport, a careful watch must be kept on:
   (a) the general condition of the patient;
   (b) the maintenance of breathing (an open airway);
   (c) the control of bleeding;
   (d) the continuous stillness of broken bones and large wounds.
(3) The transport must be safe and steady.

## Methods of carrying

If help is available, do not attempt to move a seriously ill or injured patient on your own.

### Cradle

This method is used for patients of light weight, or for children. Lift the patient by passing one of your arms well beneath his two knees and the other around his neck.

### Human crutch

Standing at his injured side, except when there is injury to an arm, assist the patient by putting your arm around his waist, grasping his clothing at his hip, and placing his arm around your neck, holding his hand with your free hand (Fig. 14.1).

If his upper arms are uninjured, and his other hand is free, the patient may gain additional help from a piece of bamboo or a walking stick.

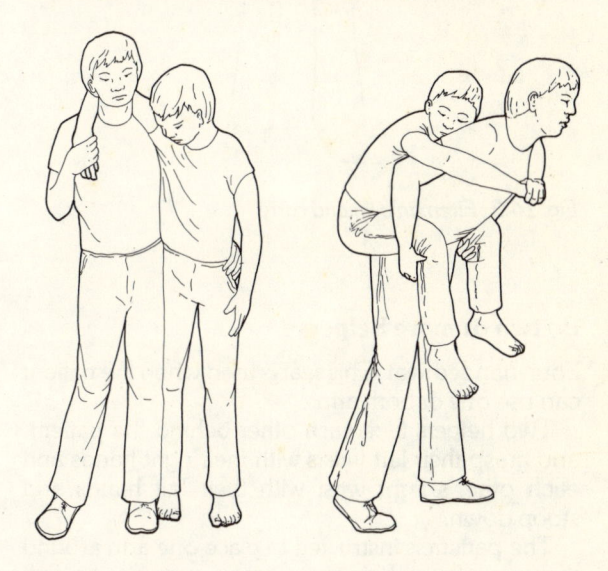

*Fig. 14.1 Human crutch*    *Fig. 14.2 Pick-a-back*

### Pick-a-back

If the patient is conscious and able to hold on, he may be carried in the ordinary pick-a-back fashion (Fig. 14.2).

### Fireman's lift and carry

Help the patient to rise to the upright position. Grasp his right wrist with your left hand. Bend down with your head under his extended right arm so that your right shoulder is level with the lower part of his belly, and place your right arm between or round his legs. Taking the weight on your right shoulder rise to the erect position. Pull the patient across both shoulders and transfer his right wrist to your right hand, so leaving your left hand free (Fig. 14.3).

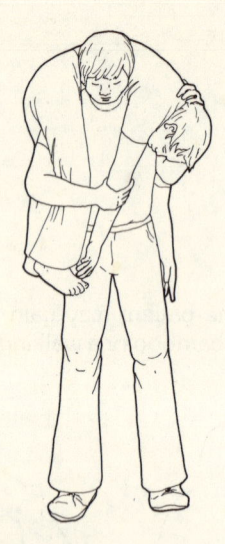

*Fig. 14.3 Fireman's lift and carry*

## By two or more helpers

Four-handed seat. This seat is used when the patient can use one or both arms.

Two helpers face each other behind the patient, and grasp their left wrists with their right hands and each other's right wrist with their left hands and stoop down.

The patient is instructed to place one arm around the neck of each helper, so that he may raise himself to sit on their hands and steady himself during transport.

The helpers rise together and step off with outside feet and walk with ordinary paces forward (Fig. 14.4).

## Two-handed seat

This seat is mostly used to carry a patient who is unable to assist by using his arms (Fig. 14.5).

Two helpers face each other and stoop, one on each side of the patient. Each helper passes his forearm nearest the patient's body under his back just below the shoulders and, if possible, takes hold of clothing. They raise the patient's back slightly and then pass their other forearms under the middle of his thighs and clasp their hands, the helper on the left of the patient with his palm upwards and holding a folded handkerchief to prevent injury by the fingernails, the helper on the right of the patient with his palms downwards (hook-grip).

The helpers rise together and step off with outside feet.

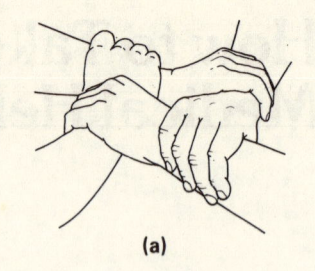

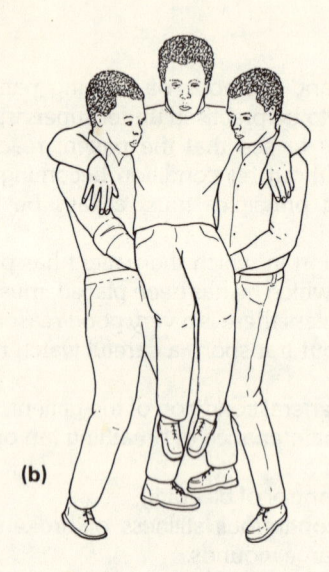

*Fig. 14.4 Four-handed seat showing (a) the wrist grasp, and (b) the carry*

## Kitchen chair method

When a patient, conscious and without serious injuries, is to be moved up or down stairs or along passageways, an ordinary kitchen-type chair can be used. The way should first of all be cleared of furniture or other obstruction.

The patient should be seated on the chair and supported by helpers, front and rear. The chair and the patient are then slowly tilted backwards and lifted.

*Taking a Patient to Medical Help* 87

supporting a back and front leg of the chair (Fig. 14.6).

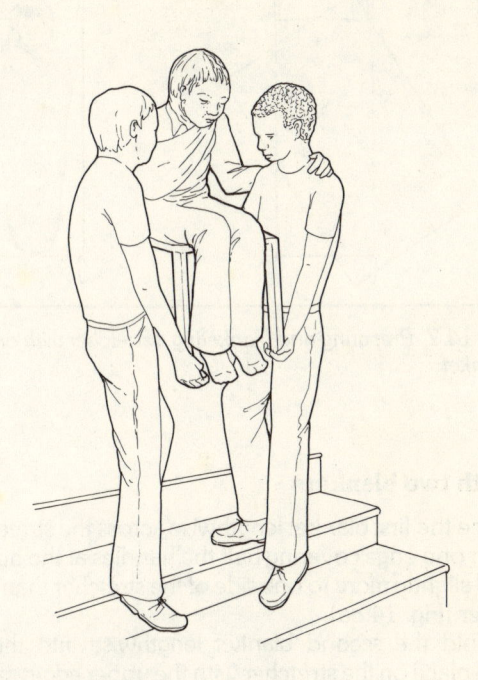

*Fig. 14.6 The kitchen chair method*

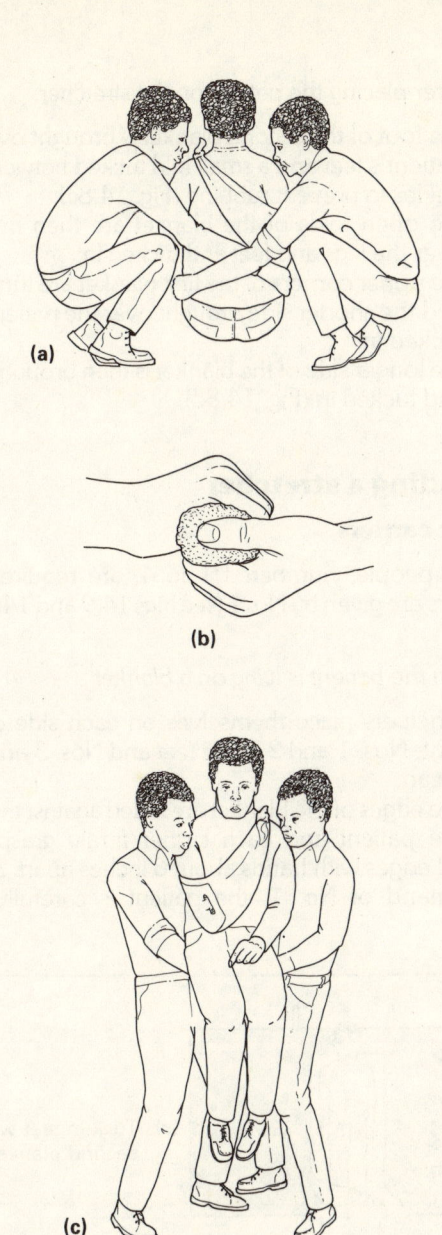

*Fig. 14.5 Two-handed seat showing (a) supporting the patient, (b) the hand clasp and (c) the carry*

One helper should support the back of the chair and the patient; the other, facing the patient, should hold the chair by the front legs and move carefully backwards down the stairs.

If the stairs or passageway are wide enough, the helpers can stand at the sides of the chair, each supporting a back and front leg of the chair (Fig. 14.6).

## Preparing and blanketing a stretcher

If you have a stretcher available:

Two helpers open and secure the stretcher. The stretcher is then tested by one person lying on it and the two ends of the stretcher raised off the ground in turn, to ensure it will take the weight of the patient. Then the stretcher is blanketed according to the number of blankets available.

### With one blanket

- Place the blanket diagonally over the stretcher.
- After placing the patient on the stretcher:
  - carry the point of the blanket round his neck and onto his chest;
  - the point of the blanket at the foot is brought up over the patient's feet and a small fold tucked between the ankles to prevent rubbing;
  - the right side of the blanket is carried over the patient and tucked in;
  - the left side of the blanket is brought over and tucked in (Fig. 14.7).

## 88  First Aid

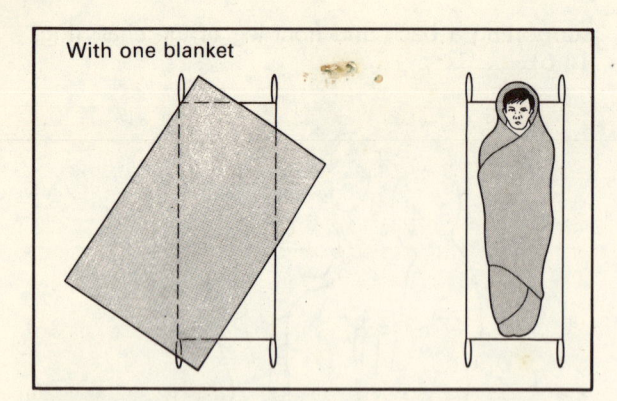

*Fig. 14.7 Preparing and blanketing a stretcher with one blanket*

### With two blankets

Place the first blanket lengthwise across the stretcher with one edge covering half the handles at the head, and slightly more to one side of the stretcher than the other (Fig. 14.8a).

Fold the second blanket lengthwise into three, and place on the stretcher with the upper edge about 15 inches below the upper side of the first blanket. Open out the folds at the lower end for about 2 feet (Fig. 14.8b).

After placing the patient on the stretcher:

- the foot of the second blanket is brought over the patient's feet and a small fold tucked between the ankles to prevent rubbing (Fig. 14.8c);
- the open folds of the blanket are then brought over the legs and feet and tucked in;
- the upper corners of the first blanket are turned in and the shorter side brought over the patient and tucked in;
- the longer side of the blanket is then brought over and tucked in (Fig. 14.8d).

## Loading a stretcher

### Four carriers

Four people, numbered 1 to 4, are required. All orders are given by No. 1 (see Figs 14.9 and 14.10).

*When the patient is lying on a blanket*

The helpers place themselves on each side of the patient; Nos. 1 and 2 at the feet and Nos. 3 and 4 at the head.

The edges of the blanket are rolled against the side of the patient and each carrier firmly grasps the rolled edges with hands about 6 inches apart. At the command of No. 1, the patient is carefully and

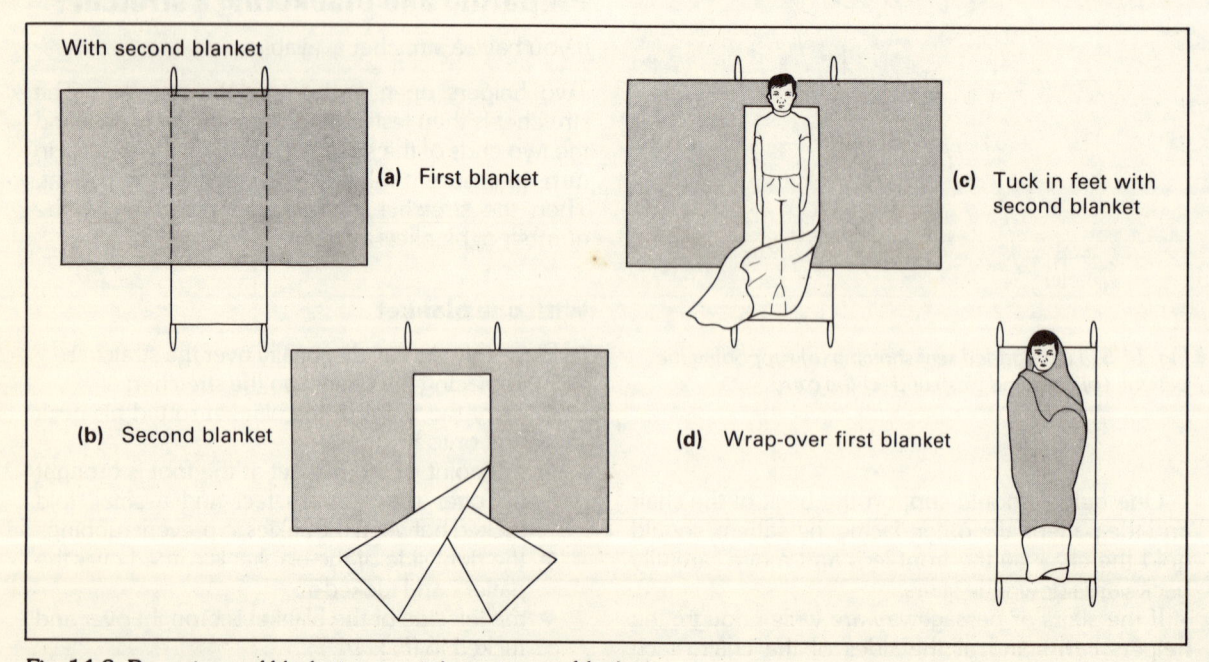

*Fig. 14.8 Preparing and blanketing a stretcher using two blankets*

(a) First blanket
(b) Second blanket
(c) Tuck in feet with second blanket
(d) Wrap-over first blanket

evenly lifted and (unless a fifth person is available to slide the stretcher under the patient), the four carriers will move with short even side-steps until the patient is directly over the canvas bed. He is then gently lowered on to it.

*When the patient is not lying on a blanket but one is available (see Fig. 14.9)*

The patient should be placed on the blanket and then lifted on to the stretcher as described above.

*When the patient is not lying on a blanket and none is available* (Fig. 14.10)

When the patient is ready for loading on to the stretcher, Nos. 2, 3 and 4 will place themselves on the left of the patient (Fig. 14.10a):

- No. 2 facing the knees;
- No. 3 facing the hips; and
- No. 4 facing the shoulders.

No. 1 will place himself on the right of the patient facing No. 3.

All will go down on their left knees and place their forearms beneath the patient, paying particular attention to the area of the injury. Using the hook-grip, No. 1 joins his left hand with the left hand of No. 4 and his right hand with the right hand of No. 3. No. 4 supports the head and shoulders, No. 2 the lower limbs (Fig. 14.10b).

When No. 1 gives the order: 'Lift', the patient must be lifted gently, slowly, and evenly, and placed on the knees of Nos. 2, 3 and 4. No. 1 will go and get the prepared stretcher and place it under the patient, so that when he is lowered on to it his head will just be clear of the top and will rest on the pillow. No. 1 will then go back to his position and rejoin hands with carriers Nos. 4 and 3 (Fig. 14.10c).

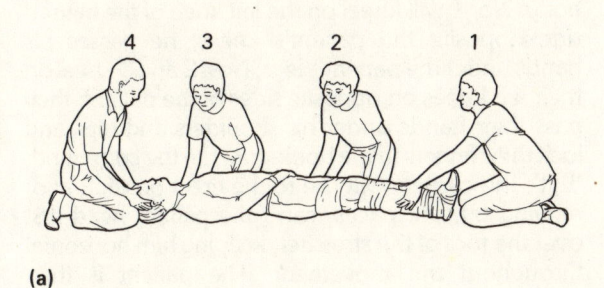

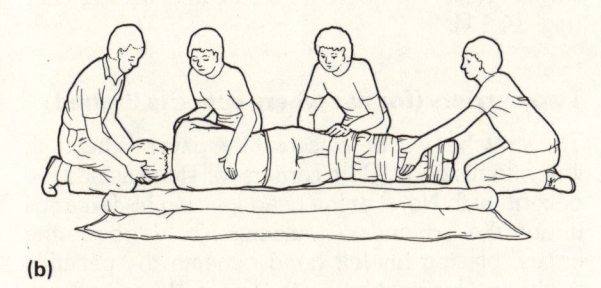

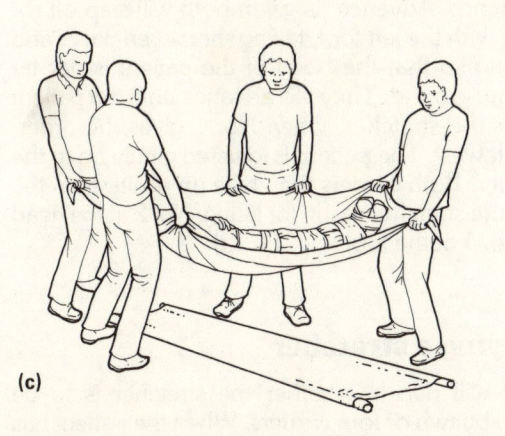

*Fig. 14.9 The blanket lift showing (a) preparation, (b) rolling the patient onto the blanket and (c) lifting the patient*

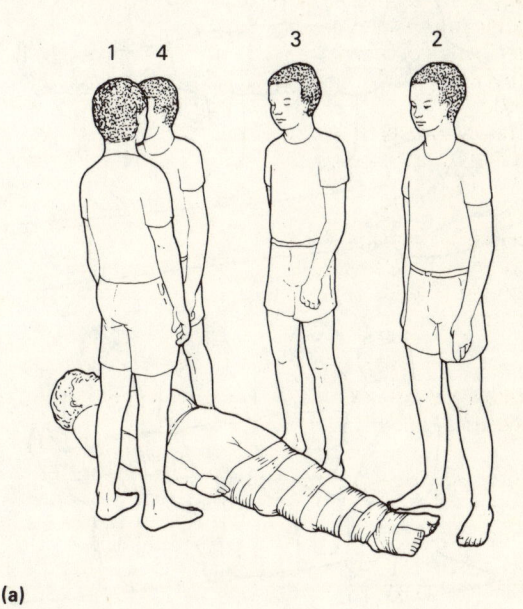

*Fig. 14.10(a) Loading a stretcher without a blanket showing position of carriers. (See overleaf for Fig. 14.10b and c.)*

90  First Aid

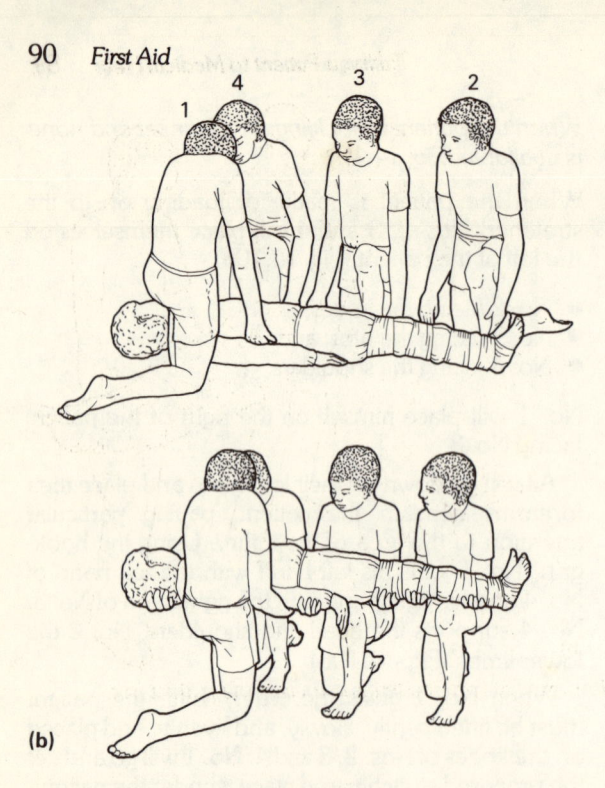

*Fig. 14.10(b) First and second moves.*

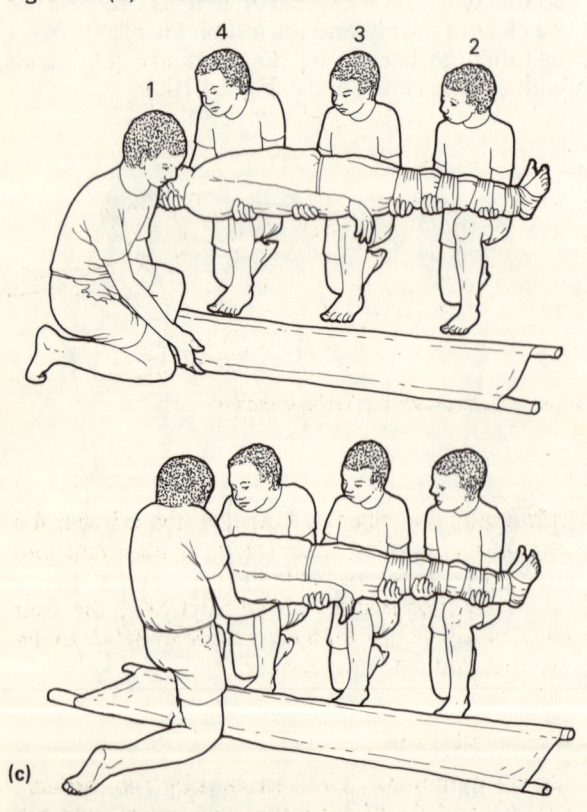

*Fig. 14.10 (c) Third and fourth moves.*

When No. 1 gives the order: 'Lower', the patient will be raised slightly from the knees of the carriers, and then lowered gently, slowly, and evenly on to the stretcher bed. The carriers then rise and turn to face the foot of the stretcher. If lifting the patient from the right side, the carriers go down on their right knees.

## Three carriers

When only three carriers are available, the stretcher will be placed at the patient's head in line with his body. No. 1 will kneel on the left knee of the injured side opposite the patient's knees; he passes his hands under the patient's legs; Nos. 2 and 3 kneel on their left knees on opposite sides of the patient; they pass their hands under his shoulders and hips and lock their fingers in the hook-grip. On the command: 'Lift', the carriers will rise to the erect position and, moving by side paces, carry the patient head first over the foot of the stretcher, keeping him horizontal throughout the movement. The patient is then lowered carefully on to the stretcher.

When unloading, the patient will be lifted and carried head foremost over the head of the stretcher (Fig. 14.11).

## Two carriers (for use where space is limited)

The stretcher will be placed at the patient's head, in line with his body. Both carriers will stand astride the patient, with No. 2 at the head, placing his forearms under the patient's shoulders, No. 1 about the knees, placing his left hand beneath the patient's thighs and his right below the knees. When both are ready, No. 1 will give the command: 'Lift'. When the command: 'Advance' is given both will step off together with the left foot, taking short even paces and stooping so that the body of the patient is not far from the ground. They will advance until the patient is over the stretcher, when No. 1 gives the order: 'Halt; lower'. The patient is lowered gently on to the stretcher. Both carriers then take up position on the left of the stretcher ready for lifting, No. 2 at the head and No. 1 at the foot (Fig. 14.12).

## Carrying a stretcher

No. 1 will decide whether the stretcher is to be carried by two or four carriers. When the patient has been placed on the stretcher, the carriers will take up their positions alongside the stretcher:

Taking a Patient to Medical Help 91

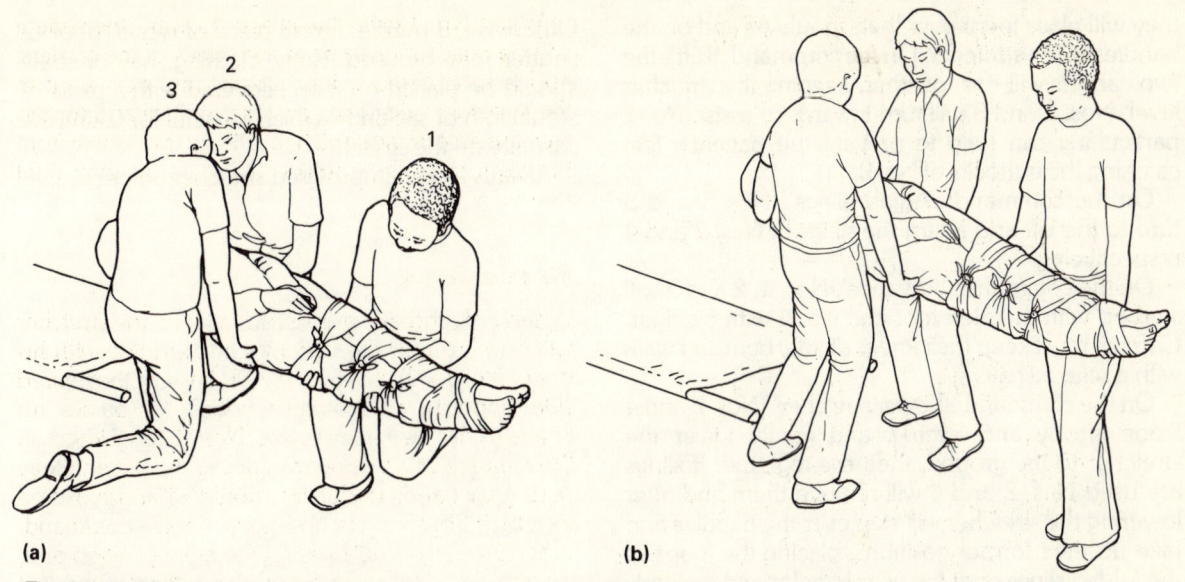

*Fig. 14.11 The three-carrier lift: (a) position of kneeling carriers and (b) carriers standing up with the patient in a horizontal position.*

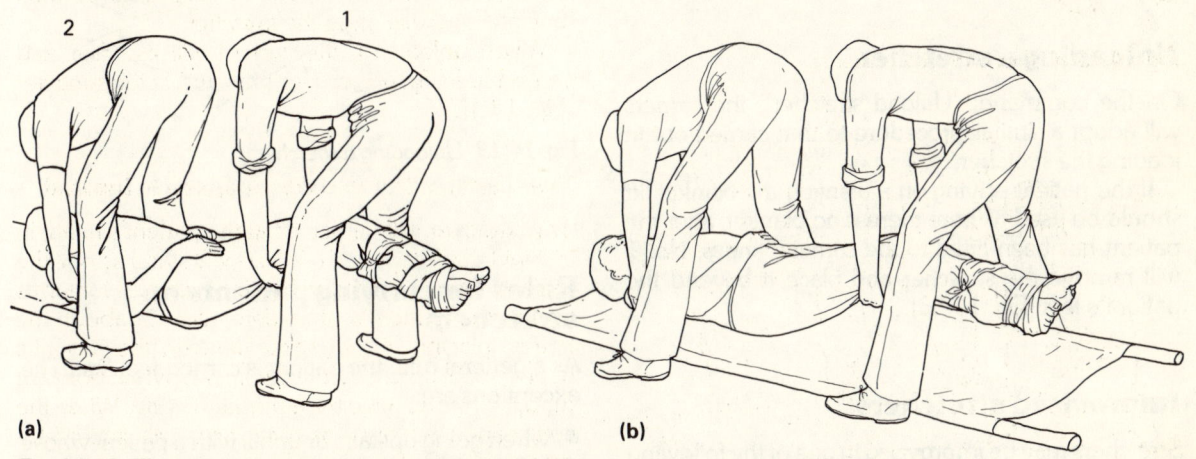

*Fig. 14.12 The two-carrier lift: (a) carrying the patient and (b) lowering the patient onto the stretcher*

- No. 1 at the foot of the stretcher on the right;
- No. 2 at the foot of the stretcher on the left;
- No. 3 at the head of the stretcher on the right;
- No. 4 at the head of the stretcher on the left.

## By four carriers

On the command: 'Hand carriage by four carriers', all four carriers will stoop together and grasp the handles with their inner hands. On the command: 'Lift', the carriers will rise together, holding the stretcher at the full extent of their arms. At the command: 'Advance', all carriers step off with the inner foot, keeping their knees slightly bent and walking with a relaxed gait.

On the command: 'Lower stretcher', the four carriers will stoop, gently lower the stretcher to the ground, and then rise together.

## By two carriers

On the command: 'Hand carriage by two carriers', Nos. 2 and 4 will then take side paces over the handles of the stretcher and, if slings are to be used, they will place them over their shoulders and on the handles of the stretcher. On the command: 'Lift', the two carriers will rise together, keeping the stretcher level. Nos. 1 and 3 will turn inwards to assist. No. 1 particularly can help to prevent the patient's feet catching the buttocks of No. 2.

On the command: 'Adjust slings', Nos. 1 and 3 turn to the left and adjust the slings of Nos. 2 and 4 respectively.

On the command: 'Advance', Nos. 1, 2 and 3 will step off with their left foot and No. 4 with his right. Carriers must keep their knees slightly bent and walk with a relaxed gait.

On the command: 'Lower stretcher', Nos. 2 and 4 stoop slowly and evenly, and gently lower the stretcher to the ground, then rise together. If slings are used Nos. 2 and 4 will remove them and after lowering the stretcher will step over the handles and take up their former positions, placing the loops of the folded slings over the near handles and the ends over the other handles.

## Unloading a stretcher

On the command: 'Unload stretcher', the carriers will adopt a similar procedure to that carried out in loading the stretcher.

If the patient is lying on a blanket, the blanket lift should be used. Where there is no blanket, after the patient has been lifted to the carriers' knees, No. 1 will remove the stretcher and place it beyond the patient's feet (Fig. 14.13).

## Improvised stretchers

Stretchers may be improvised in one of the following ways:

(1) Turn the sleeves of two or three coats inside out; pass two strong poles or bamboos through them. Button the coats. The poles may be kept apart by strips of wood lashed to the poles at both ends of the 'bed' formed by the coats (Fig. 14.14).
(2) Make holes in the bottom corners of one or more sacks and pass strong poles through them, keeping them apart as above.
(3) Tie broad bandages at intervals to two strong poles.
(4) Spread out a rug, piece of sacking, tarpaulin or a strong blanket, and roll up two strong poles in the sides.

Otherwise, a hurdle, broad piece of wood, door or shutter may be used. Rugs, clothing, hay or straw should be placed on it and covered with a piece of stout cloth or sacking—which is useful for taking the casualty off the stretcher.

Always test an improvised stretcher before use.

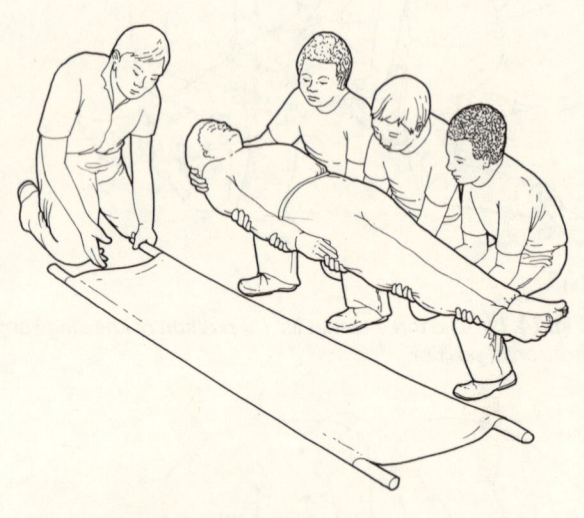

*Fig. 14.13 Unloading a stretcher*

## Rules for carrying patients on stretchers

As a general rule, the patient is carried feet first. The exceptions are:

- when going upstairs or uphill with a patient whose legs are uninjured;
- when going downstairs or downhill with a patient whose legs are injured;
- when carrying a patient to the side or foot of a bed;
- when loading a motor vehicle.

### To cross uneven ground

If possible the stretcher should be carried by four carriers, and kept as nearly level as possible. This can be done, and the patient prevented from falling off, by each carrier independently adjusting the height of the stretcher as necessary. Over very uneven ground for a short distance, the four carriers should face inwards.

*Taking a Patient to Medical Help* 93

With two sticks 2 metres long and two shirts

Stretcher

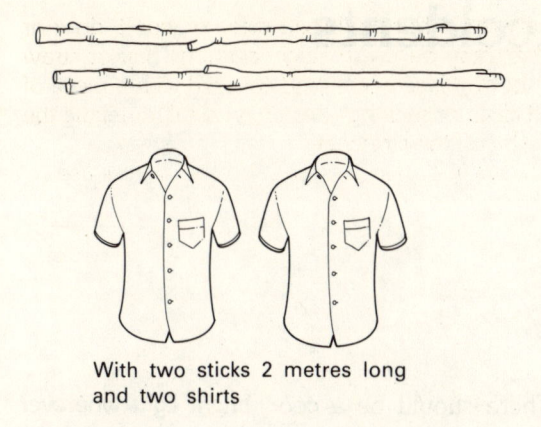

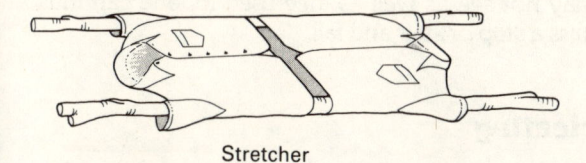

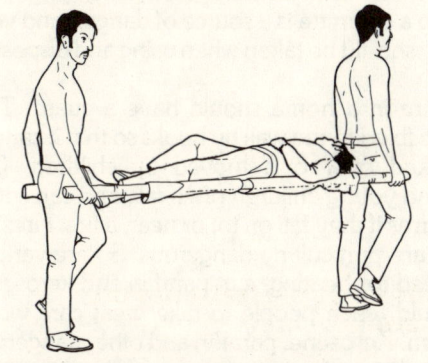

In this way it will be possible to carry the patient comfortably to the hospital or the health centre.

*Fig. 14.14 Improvising a stretcher*

## To cross a ditch or stream

The stretcher is lowered near the edge of the ditch. The two front carriers get into the ditch and all four carriers lift the stretcher together, moving it forward until the rear handles rest on the edge of the ditch. The rear carriers get into the ditch and the stretcher is then moved forward on to the ground, and rests there while the rear carriers get out of the ditch.

## To cross a wall

Avoid crossing a wall, if possible, even if it means a longer distance. If there is no gap, the stretcher is lifted on to the wall so that the front runners are just over it, and the stretcher held level by the rear carriers while the front carriers cross the wall. All carriers then lift together and the stretcher is moved forward until the rear carriers are clear of the wall, the stretcher being held level by the carriers in front. The remaining carriers then cross the wall and the stretcher is lowered carefully from the wall. The stretcher is then carried in the usual way.

Using a stretcher properly is a fairly complicated procedure and frequent practice under knowledgeable supervision is essential.

# Appendix I. How to Prevent Accidents and Poisonings

An accident can cripple or even kill. It is important, therefore, for all of us to do everything we can to see that houses, gardens, compounds, land, roads, shops, factories, fields and schools—in fact, all the places where people live, work or pass by—are as safe as possible.

## Floors

Floors should be even and flat. When they have bumps and holes in them they are dangerous and can cause falls. Fill in holes as soon as they appear and patch any torn linoleum so that the surface is quite smooth. Holes and frayed edges of carpets, rugs and mats should be mended as soon as they appear. See that all rugs and carpets are also flat and do not slip about when they are walked on.

## Furniture

Old nails and bits of splintered wood sticking out from furniture—tables, beds, chairs and cupboards—can cause nasty cuts and, if germs get into them, can result in serious illness. So remove or knock in any such nails, and sandpaper any rough or splintered furniture.

## Lights

All lights (except electric light bulbs) need to be well guarded. Lamps and candles should be placed on a very firm base: they can be knocked over very easily and cause a fire. Sometimes young children try to touch a naked flame, and get burned that way. Candles and lamps should be stood out of draughts and away from curtains, screens or mosquito netting. If they have to be carried while alight, see that they are carried very, very carefully and are fixed well in their holders.

There should be a good bright light wherever there are steps or stairs. Elderly people, especially, may not see as well as they used to, and can thus miss a step or stair and fall.

## Heating

Any lighter or match which is used for making a fire or lighting a cigarette is a source of danger, and very great care should be taken when using and disposing of it.

Each fire in a home should have a guard. This should be fixed to the wall by hooks so that it cannot be knocked over or removed by children. Old people and young children often fall, and can suffer severe burns if they fall on to, or near, a fire. Fires on the floor are particularly dangerous. So are various liquids used for heating, e.g. paraffin and kerosene. You should teach people to take great care when using them. Kerosene, paraffin and other dangerous fluids should not be stored in empty bottles which have had soft drinks in them. Children and other people may drink from them, thinking that they contain lemonade, Coca Cola or some other pleasant drink.

Cylinders and drums of gas and other fuel should be stored well away from fires.

If bonfires are lit, they should be well watched and children encouraged to play some distance away from them.

## Electric equipment and implements

People should treat all electricity and electrical goods with great respect. They can burn and kill. Each electric fire, kettle, iron or tool, if not fixed properly or if not used in the proper way, can result in fuses and burns. Plugs, switches and wires must never come into contact with water. All frayed wires should be replaced by new wires. Only someone who has learned how to do this kind of repair work properly, should do it. People who have not had any training or lessons in mending electrical goods should take all such work to an expert to do.

Electric plugs can also be dangerous if there are small children about, because they are likely to push things such as bits of wire or the prongs of a fork into them. This could mean a very nasty electric shock for them. It could even kill them.

Before pulling out a plug, the electric current should always be switched off. It should also be switched off before lifting a kettle, and before trying to unwedge a piece of toast jammed in an electric toaster.

## Cooking and meal times

Very many children get scalded because they pull cooking pots and pans over themselves. All handles should be turned so that small children cannot reach them. All pots of hot food and liquid placed on the table at meal times should be put out of the reach of babies and small children. If the table has a cloth on it, the edge of this may be pulled by a young child, thus bringing down the hot contents of a pot or dish. So it is important to watch carefully for this danger.

## Water

Metal baths containing hot water get very hot and can burn even when the water has cooled down.

People can drown in very little water; it does not have to be deep. When a child or elderly person goes to a bath, pond, river or near a pit latrine, well, water tank, swamp or spring, he should always have someone with him. This also applies to people who are mentally confused or who suffer from fits.

## Poisoning

Much can be done to prevent the swallowing of poison by mistake. All medicines, bleaches, and disinfectants should be kept well out of the reach of children and mentally ill or confused people. Particularly dangerous are:

- ammonia;
- bleaches;
- castor beans;
- caustic soda;
- detergents;
- D.D.T., lindane, sheep-dip and other insecticides;
- insect-killers;
- kerosene, gasolene, petrol and paraffin;
- matches;
- medicines, including iron pills;
- oven cleaners;
- paint restorers and strippers;
- pest poisons;
- poisonous leaves, seeds, bark, leaves, juice, berries and fruit;
- rat poison;
- soap mixtures, powders and fluids;
- tincture of iodine;
- wood alcohol.

Fluids should never be transferred from one bottle to another. It is easy to forget that a lemonade bottle has been used for strong bleaching liquid, for example, and other people will not be aware of it.

Many pesticides, as well as being poisonous, are also inflammable (they burn easily and quickly), so their use and storage should be carefully controlled and supervised. They should never be stored in an area used for cooking or serving food.

If possible, medicines should be kept in a locked cupboard or otherwise stored on a very high shelf which a child cannot reach—even when he stands on a chair or table. Many medicines and pills are brightly coloured. Children often think they are sweets and good to eat. If they do swallow them they can cause a serious illness and even death.

Fumes from charcoal fires, oil stoves, etc. are bad for people. They can slowly poison. Fresh air should blow through a house whenever possible.

Fumes from an old motor-car or motor-bicycle—especially in a closed shed or garage—can also make people very ill. All families with a motor-car or motor-bicycle should know this and take care.

## Food poisoning

There is a lot you can do to prevent people being poisoned by water or food.

Ideally, all water that does not come from a safe water system should be boiled before drinking. This is especially important for babies and small children, and at times when there are cases of diarrhoea, typhoid, hepatitis or cholera in the area.

Water from rivers and holes, even when it looks clean, can spread disease and should be boiled before use.

You should also see that people know that they should not let flies and other insects land and crawl on food. Every insect can carry disease. Dirty dishes should be washed at once, and food scraps burnt or buried. Both attract flies. All food should be stored in tins, boxes or in cupboards with one side of wire-mesh to allow some air to enter.

All fruit should be washed in clean water. Children should be taught to wash any food they drop before continuing to eat it.

It is also important to wash hands before eating or drinking, especially after defaecation (passing stools).

Only well-cooked meat should be eaten. Make certain that cooked meat—especially cooked pig—has no raw parts. Raw pork can cause very dangerous diseases.

If food is old, or smells bad, it should not be eaten as it could be poisonous. If a tin of food is swollen or the contents spurt out when you open it, do not eat that food: it is bad.

The plates, cups, knives, forks and spoons used by people with diarrhoea or any other disease should be boiled before being used by other people.

## Guns, knives and other sharp things

It is very important to see that people who have guns, including guards, policemen, soldiers and game-keepers, etc. are careful not to leave their guns and rifles lying around. Guns should always be locked up when not in use.

Cooking knives, scissors, gardening and carpentry tools can all be dangerous in the hands of children. They should be kept well out of their reach. Parents should give small children blunt-ended scissors when they want to cut up paper or help with a household task.

## Motor-cars and bicycles

Many accidents are caused by faults in motor-cars or bicycles, and by bad driving and riding.

All essential parts of motor-cars should be kept in good condition, and wheels and tyres checked regularly.

Motor-bikes and cycles should also be overhauled regularly, and all needed repairs done immediately. Saddles should be firm, and riders taught to ride properly in quiet places until they are ready to ride in traffic. A bicycle should be the right size for the person who is going to ride it.

The rules of the road should be known and practised at all times by drivers, riders and pedestrians.

People who have drunk alcohol recently should not drive a car nor ride a motor-bike or cycle.

## People who are most likely to have accidents

Until babies are at least 1 year old, they depend upon other people completely. Even then, accidents can happen to them. For example, if cloth or plastic such as clothing, cot pillow, plastic covers etc., cover a baby's nose and mouth, he will not be able to breathe and will die. Or he may choke on a piece of dry food. If he is left on the floor alone, he may roll over on to a fire if it does not have a guard. He may knock over a lamp or a candle while crawling about, or he may get a ribbon, cord or string from his clothes caught round his neck.

He may even fall off the back of his mother or an older brother or sister if they are not careful when they tie his cloth. Children have to be taught how to carry babies gently and carefully. Sometimes a baby puts his head between the bars of his cot or playpen and then is unable to pull it back again, or he may get his head into a pot or saucepan and then not be able to get it off.

When he begins to crawl, sharp stones and broken steps could cut him. Some toys have sharp edges and these should be smoothed down before being given to a child. Broken glass should be picked up and carefully disposed of whenever you see it lying around: crawling children do not know the danger of it.

### Young children

A toddler or a young child faces all these dangers and others besides! Because he can get around, he will find himself amongst other hazards. He can fall into fires, ponds, latrines, compost heaps, swamps, fish ponds, rivers and springs. This is why it is so important to keep each of these guarded or covered. A child should never be left alone in a bath. A small child will also climb tables, chairs, steps or walls. He is very likely to fall.

A young child loves to touch everything which interests him. This can mean electrical things, oil, gas, petrol, stoves, knives, tools, taps, all of which could mean danger for him. He will probably want to taste liquids in bottles, and this is why they should all be kept out of his reach for even the glass bottles containing milk or soft drinks are dangerous for a child. If he falls when he is clutching one, he may be badly cut by the broken glass.

Snakes and some animals are dangerous, of course, and crocodiles and hyenas especially so. So are some insects, fruits and berries. Children should be taught very early on in their lives which local fruits and berries can be eaten and which will make them ill.

Children also have to be taught about traffic; they must learn to look both ways before running across a road. It is also important to ensure that they can ride a bicycle well before allowing them to ride one on a busy road.

Children's toys and furniture, e.g. cots, should not be covered with lead-containing paint and small children must be carefully supervised if lead pipes, etc. are in their playing area.

## Old people

Very old people sometimes have disabilities or impairments which may lead to accidents. Many are unable to see, smell and hear as well as they could when younger; and they may forget the warnings they have been given. Sometimes they will not be able to move quickly because they are stiff from rheumatism, or crippled by arthritis. They may be breathless, or their minds may be confused.

Old people are particularly likely to become unsteady and fall. When they do, they often break a bone because bones become very fragile with age. This is why it is important to see that floors, linoleum, carpeting, rugs and mats are safe and that there is a good light over all steps and stairs. If it is possible to avoid it, they should not be given open lights such as lamps and candles to carry. Torches are much better as there is no risk of fire from them.

If an elderly person wears shoes or sandals, they should fit well and not be worn or torn. If their shoes or boots have laces to them they should be firmly tied so that they do not come undone while they are walking.

## Others

People who are crippled, mentally disabled or confused, blind or deaf will also need special protection from hazards and dangers which may cause them to have accidents.

So will women when they are pregnant; because of their swollen bellies they sometimes have poor balance and fall easily.

# Appendix II. How to Use some of the Medicines Mentioned in this Book

| Name of medicine | Mainly for treatment of | How to give it | Baby less than 1 year old | Small child from 1 to 3 years | Child from 4 to 12 years | Adult or child over 12 years old |
|---|---|---|---|---|---|---|
| **Aspirin** | Fever and pains | 500 mg tablets | — | ¼ | ½ | 1 to 3 |
|  |  |  | ← Three times a day → |  |  |  |
| **Atropine** | Abdominal pains | Intramuscular injection | — | — | — | ¼ mg; repeat once if necessary |
| **Aureomycin** (eye ointment) | Eye diseases | Ointment | Put a little ointment in the corner of the eye two or three times a day for 3–5 days. |  |  |  |
| **Belladonna tincture** | Abdominal pains | Drops in a glass of water | — | Three drops per year of age, but no more than 30 drops |  | 30 drops |
| **Ergotamine** | Bleeding after delivery or miscarriage | 1 mg tablets | — | — | — | One or two; repeat once or twice if necessary |
| **Gentian violet** or **tincture of iodine** | Cleaning wounds | Liquid to put on skin | First wash the skin with soap and water, leave to dry, then put the liquid on the skin with a clean cloth |  |  |  |
| **Iron sulphate** | Weakness, tiredness | 250 mg tablets | — | — | One to be taken with food twice a day for 1 month |  |
| **Oral rehydration salts** | Diarrhoea | One packet dissolved in 1 litre of drinking water | As much as is needed to quench thirst; then one or two cupfuls for each watery stool passed; adults may need several litres a day. Continue until diarrhoea stops |  |  |  |
| **Oxytocine** | Expulsion of placenta; to stop bleeding *quickly* after delivery or miscarriage | Intramuscular injection ampoules of 5 I.U. (international units) | — | — | — | One intramuscular injection of contents of a 5 I.U. ampoule |
| **Procaine penicillin** (aqueous solution) | Infections | Intramuscular injection | — | 250,000 units | 500,000 units | 1,000,000 units |
|  |  |  |  | ← Every day for 3 days → |  |  |
| **Phenobarbital** | To treat someone who has convulsions | 50 mg tablets | — | ½ | 1 | 1 to 2 |
|  |  |  |  | Two or three times a day for 2 days; then half the dosage for 6 months |  |  |
| **Sulphadiazine** | Infections | 500 mg tablets | ½ | 1 | 2 | 3 |
|  |  |  | To be taken with a glass of water four times a day for 3 days |  |  |  |
| **Tetracycline** | Infections | 250 mg tablets | ⅕ | ½ | 1 | 1 to 3 |
|  |  |  | ← Four times a day for 3 days → |  |  |  |

# Appendix III. How to Teach what is in this Book

Addresses from which Teaching Materials can be obtained

| | |
|---|---|
| Teaching Aids at Low Cost (TALC),<br>Institute of Child Health,<br>30 Guilford Street,<br>London, WC1N 1EH, England. | Slide sets, weight charts, aids to weight charts (flannelgraphs, etc.) Free booklist, English, French and Spanish. |
| Courtejoie, Dr. J.<br>Centre pour le Promotion de la Santé,<br>Kangu Majumbe, République de Zaire. | Excellent simple material for villages in French, some English, and local languages. |
| Voluntary Health Association of India (C.A.H.P.)<br>045, South Extension, Part II,<br>New Delhi, 110049, India. | Flannelgraphs, books, flip charts, etc. List available. Material in English and local languages. |
| Christian Medical College and Hospital,<br>Vellore 4,<br>Madras, India. | Posters, flash cards, flannelgraphs in English and local languages. |
| F.A.O.,<br>Nutrition and Home Economic Division,<br>Rome, Italy. | Wide variety of material, some useful at village level. English, French and Spanish. |
| W.H.O.<br>Geneva, Switzerland. | Material in English, French and Spanish. |
| Health Education Department,<br>Addis Ababa, Ethiopia. | Teaching kits. Material in English and some local languages. |
| International Development Research Centre (I.R.D.C.)<br>P.O. Box 8500<br>Ottawa, Canada, K19 3HG. | Booklets on China. Also on the place of doctors and auxiliaries in health care. Free to those in poorer countries. |
| National Food and Nutrition Commission,<br>P.O. Box 2669,<br>Lusaka, Zambia. | Posters and teaching material on nutrition, English and local languages. |
| Chief Education Officer,<br>Public Health Department,<br>Ministry of Health,<br>Ibadan, Nigeria. | Posters and material in English and main Nigerian languages. |
| Matériel Réalisé à l'Atelier de Matériel Didactique,<br>Busiga, B.P.18,<br>Ngozi, Burundi. | Good flip charts; a teaching plan using flip charts in French and local languages. |

| | |
|---|---|
| World Neighbours,<br>5116 North Portland Avenue,<br>Oklahoma City,<br>Oklahoma 73112, U.S.A. | Filmstrips, manuals, flip charts in English, French and Spanish. |
| Shanta Bhawan Community Health Programme<br>Box 252,<br>Kathmandu, Nepal. | Slides, flip charts. |
| Carlos Campesino,<br>Apartado 2444,<br>Guatemala City, Guatemala | Battery-powered projectors and film strip sets. |
| O.C.E.A.C.,<br>B.P. 288,<br>Yaounde, Cameroun. | Material in French. |
| Health Education Supply Centre,<br>P.O. Box 922,<br>Loma Linda,<br>California 92354, U.S.A. | Books (hard and soft covers) and visual aids. |
| The Philippine Lutheran Church,<br>P.O. Box 507,<br>Manila, Philippines, D404. | Flip charts. |
| Saidpur Concern, Teaching Aids Workshop,<br>c/o Concern, P.O. Box 650,<br>Dacca, Bangladesh. | Flip charts. |
| I.L.O.,<br>Geneva, Switzerland. | Booklets on use of the flannelgraph, etc. |
| I.T.D.G.,<br>Parnell House, Wilton Road,<br>London, SW1, England. | Booklets on simple technology; will send advice on technical problems. |
| V.I.T.A.,<br>3706 Rhode Island Avenue,<br>Mt. Rainier,<br>Maryland 20822, U.S.A. | Village equipment handbook. |
| ENI Communication Centre,<br>P.O. Box 2361,<br>Addis Ababa, Ethiopia. | Education packages and visual aids in child health and nutrition. |
| African Medical and Research Foundation,<br>Wilson Airport, P.O. Box 30125,<br>Nairobi, Kenya. | Booklets for auxiliaries. |
| American Foundation for Overseas Blind, Inc.,<br>22 West 17th Street,<br>New York,<br>New York 10011, U.S.A. | Material on blindness from lack of vitamin A. |
| Alfalit Boliviano,<br>Junin 6305, Casilla 1466,<br>Cochabamba, Bolivia. | Simple booklets on health in Spanish and English. |

## Appendix III

Centro Andino de Comunicaciones,
Casilla 2774,
Cochabamba, Bolivia.

Flip charts in Spanish.

Nutrition Center of the Philippines,
Communications Department,
Nichols Interchange,
South Superhighway,
Makati, Rizal, Philippines.

Leaflets and fact sheets in English.

The Nutrition Section,
Public Health Department,
P.O. Box 2084,
Konedobu, Papua New Guinea.

Posters and booklets.

# Index

Abdomen
  acute, 42–4
  wounds, 20
  see also Gut
Abortion, 49–51
Accidents
  determining severity, 2
  groups most at risk, 96–7
  history, 1
  prevention, 94–7
Acid damage to eye, 82
Acute abdomen, 42–4
Airway
  clearing, 8, 9
  obstruction, causes of, 9
  see also Breathing
Alcohol, effect on pain, 5
Alkali damage to eye, 82
Allergic shock, 24
Ammonia poisoning, 33
Anaemia
  during pregnancy, 48
  severe, 51
Angina, 16
Ankle, fractures, 79
Antibiotics, possible risks, 24
Antihistamine poisoning, 33
Antitoxins, possible risks, 24
Appendicitis, 42–3
Arms, fractures, 76–7
Arsenic poisoning, 34
Arteries, 3
  bleeding from, 17–18
Artificial respiration, 10–11
Aspirin
  poisoning, 33
  use and dosage, 98
Asthma, acute attacks, 13
Atropine, use and dosage, 98
Aureomycin, use and dosage, 98

Babies, see Childbirth; Pregnancy
Bandages and bandaging, 22–3
  emergency dressings, 23
  of fractures, 71–2
Battery acid poisoning, 33
Belladonna, use and dosage, 98
Belly pain, see Stomach ache
Bites, causing respiratory arrest, 7
  see also Dog bites; Snake bites; Spider bites
Black magic, loss of consciousness due to, 29

Bladder, 3
  catheterisation, 45–6
  stones, 44
Bleeding
  arterial, 17–18
  behind cornea, 81
  capillary, 17
  during pregnancy, 49–51, 52
  estimating blood loss, 22
  excessive, 2
  from ear, 82
  from nose, 83
  from palm of hand, 22
  from tongue or cheek, 84
  from tooth socket, 84
  in white of eye, 82
  internal, 5, 6
  venous, 17
Blood circulation, 3
Bones, see Fractures; Musculo-skeletal system
Bowel, 3
Brain damage, 73–4
  cause of fits, 5
  malaria of the brain, 65
Breast abscess, 60–1
Breast bone, fractured, 76
Breast-feeding, 61
Breathing
  arrest, 9–11
  artificial respiration, 10–11
  difficulties, 9–16
    signs and symptoms, 9–10
    treatment, 10–11
  during fits, 5
  establishment in newborn baby, 58
  observation, 4, 9
  restoring, 2
  see also Airway; Respiration
Burns and scalds, 6, 26–8
  accident prevention measures, 94–5
  chemical, 28
  depth, 26
  electrical burns, 28
  extent, 26
  minor, 28
  treatment, 26–7

Capillaries
  bleeding from, 17
  see also Vascular system

Cardiac emergencies, see Heart
Cardio-pulmonary arrest, 2
  priority actions, 5
Cardio-pulmonary system, 3
Catheter, insertion, 45, 46
Caustic soda poisoning, 33
Cheek, bleeding from, 84
Chemical burns, 28
Chest
  compression, 7
  wounds, 20, 21–2
Childbirth, 6, 53–61
  abnormal presentations, 58
  delivery, 55–8
  hypothermia of the newborn, 68
  immediate care of baby, 58–9
  premature, 54, 60
  preparation of mother, 55
  problems of urinating after, 45
  signs of congenital problems, 60
  signs of onset of labour, 54–5
  signs of special risk, 53
  stages of labour, 53–4
  tears to vagina, 60
  tetanus in newborn baby, 62–3
  see also Pregnancy
Choking, 11–13
Clavicle, see Collar bone
Cold, problems of, 68–9
  frostbite, 69
  hypothermia, 68–9
Collar bone, fractured, 76
Coma, 6
  insulin and diabetic, comparison, 30
Concussion, loss of consciousness due to, 30–1
Consciousness
  during fits, 5
  levels of, 4
  loss of, treatment, 29–31
Constipation, during pregnancy, 49
Convulsions, see Fits
Corneal ulcers, 81
Cradle, as means of transport, 85
Cramps, heat, 67
Cuts
  closing, 19
  stitching, 19–20
  see also Wounds

Deformity through injury, 5

# Index

Dehydration
  causing fits, 65–6
  tests, 40
  see also Fluid replacement
Diabetes mellitus, loss of consciousness due to, 30
Diarrhoea
  and dehydration, 65–6
  avoidance of dehydration, 40–1
Digestive system, 3
Discharges from orifices, 5
Dog bites, 38
Drowning, 13
Drugs, effect on pain, 5
Drunkenness, loss of consciousness due to, 29–30

Ear
  bleeding from, 82
  foreign body in, 83
ECM, see External cardiac massage (ECM)
Electrical burns, 28
Electrical equipment, accident prevention measures, 94–5
Electrocution, cause of respiratory arrest, 7
Emergencies
  initial action, 2–3
  nature and severity, 2
  sudden illness, 3
Epilepsy, as cause of fits, 5, 65
Ergotamine, use and dosage, 98
Examination of patient
  checks on parts of body, 3
  order, 2
Excretory system, 3
External cardiac massage (ECM), 14–15
Eyes
  acid/alkali damage, 82
  common problems, 81
  foreign body in, 82
  inflammation from cobra venom, 35
  injuries, 82
  irritation by ammonia, 33
  see also Pupils of eyes

Facial bones, fractures, 74
Fainting, 29
Femur, fractures, 79
Fever, causing fits, 62
Fibula, fractures, 79
Fingers, fractures, 77
Fireman's lift and carry, 85–6
First aid
  assessing need, 1–2
  order of care, 1
  priority actions, 6
  purpose, 1
Fits, 6, 62–6
  causes, 62
    dehydration, 65–6
    epilepsy, 5, 65
    high fever, 62
    meningitis, 64–5
    tetanus, 62–4
  during pregnancy, 52, 62
  following brain damage, 73
  immediate treatment, 62
Floors, accident prevention measures, 94
Fluid replacement, 6, 8, 27, 41, 66
  see also Rehydration fluid
Follow-up care, 8
Food poisoning, 32
  accident prevention measures, 95–6
  compared with metal poisoning, 34
  from shell-fish, 37
Foot, fractures, 80
Foreign body
  in ear, 83
  in eye, 82
  in nose, 83
Four-handed seat, 86
Fractures, 70–80
  ankle, 79
  arm, 76–7
  breast bone, 76
  classification, 70
  collar bone, 76
  facial bones, 74
  foot bones, 80
  general first aid, 80
  greenstick, 70
  jaw, 74
  leg, 79
  pelvis, 78
  ribs, 77–8
  shoulder blade, 78–9
  skull, 72–4
  spine, 74–6
  symptoms, 70–1
  transport to hospital, 75–6
  treatment, 71
Frostbite, 69
Furniture, accident prevention measures, 94

Gall-bladder, 3
Gangrene
  from frostbite, 69
  gas, 25
Gas poisoning, 34
Genito-urinary system, 3
  acute conditions, 44–6
Gentian violet, use and dosage, 98
Glaucoma, 81
Gonorrhoea, 45
Greenstick fracture, 70
Gunshot wounds, 20
  accident prevention measures, 96
Gut
  acute abdomen, 42–4
  blockage, 42–3

Haemorrhoids, see Piles (haemorrhoids)
Hand, bleeding from palm, 22
Heart, 3
  cardiac arrest, 14
  cardio-pulmonary arrest, 2, 5
  emergencies, 13–16
  external cardiac massage, 14–15
  function, 2
  massage for infants, 15
  see also Pulse rate
Heart attack, 6, 16
  loss of consciousness due to, 31
Heat, problems of, 67–8
  cramps, 67
  exhaustion, 67
  stroke, 6, 67–8
Heating appliances, accident prevention measures, 94
Hip, fractures, 78
History
  of accident or illness, 1
  of patient, 2
  passing to supervisor, 7–8
Hot compresses, 24, 25
Human crutch, as means of transport, 85
Humerus, fractures, 76–7
Hypothermia, 68–9
Hysteria, loss of consciousness due to, 29

Illness, sudden, checks in cases of, 3
  see also Emergencies; First aid
Indigestion, during pregnancy, 47
Infection
  after stitching wound, 20
  causes of, 23
  treatment, 24–5
Information, see History
Injuries
  checklist for treatment, 6
  determining severity, 2
  see also Wounds

# Index

Insecticide poisoning, 33
Insulin injections, 30
Iodine, use and dosage, 98
Iritis, 81
Iron, use and dosage, 98
Iron poisoning, 34

Jaw, fractured, 74
Jelly-fish stings, 37

Kidney stones, 44
Kidneys, see Genito-urinary system
Kitchen chair method of transport, 86–7
Knee-cap, fractures, 79
Knee reflexes, test for tetanus, 64
Knife wounds, 20
Knives
   accident prevention measures, 96
   wounds, 20

Lead poisoning, 34
Leg, fractures, 79
Lightning strikes, 69
Lights, accident prevention measures, 94
Liver, 3
Lungs, 3
   damage from fractured ribs, 77–8
   function, 2
Lysol poisoning, 34

Malaria of the brain, 65
Malnutrition, during pregnancy, 48
Medicines causing allergic shock, 24
Meningitis, fits caused by, 64–5
Mercury poisoning, 34
Motor vehicles, accident prevention measures, 96
Mouth
   bleeding from tongue or cheek, 84
   bleeding from tooth socket, 84
Movement, degree of ability, 5
Mucus, discharge, 5
Musculo-skeletal system, 3
   sprains, 80
   strains, 80
   see also Fractures

Nausea, 5
   during pregnancy, 47
Neck, compression, 7
Nerves, controlling breathing, 9

Nose
   bleeding, 83
   foreign body, 83
   fracture, 74
Numbness, 5

Observation of patient, 1
   in heart emergencies, 13–14
   of breathing difficulties, 7
   of poisoning, 32
Oxygen deficiency, cause of respiratory arrest, 9
Oxytocine, use and dosage, 98

Pain
   inside eye, 81
   observation, 4–5
Pallor, 4
Paraffin poisoning, 34
Paralysis, 5
   cause of respiratory arrest, 9
Paraquat poisoning, 34
Patella, see Knee-cap
Pelvis, see Hip
Penicillin
   allergic shock, 24
   use and dosage, 98
Peritonitis, 43, 44
Petrol poisoning, 34
Phenobarbital, use and dosage, 98
Pick-a-back, as means of transport, 85
Piles (haemorrhoids), during pregnancy, 49
Poisoning, 32–9
   accident prevention measures, 95
   antidotes, 33
   by acids, 33
   by alkalis, 33
   by antihistamines, 33
   by aspirin, 33
   by inhalation, 34
   by insecticides, 33
   by iron, 34
   by jelly-fish stings, 37
   by lead, 34
   by lysol, 34
   by mercury, 34
   by paraffin and petrol, 34
   by plants, 34–5
   by scorpion stings, 36–7
   by sedatives, 33
   by snake bites, 35–6
   by spider bites, 37
   by weedkillers, 34
   cause of fits, 5
   cause of respiratory arrest, 7

   checks for, 2
   food, 32, 34, 95–6
   from piercing by fish, 38
   priority actions, 6
   routes, 32
   symptoms, 32
   through skin, 34
Pregnancy
   anaemia and malnutrition, 48
   avoidance of illness, 47
   danger signs, 49–52
   ectopic, 50
   indigestion, 47
   low back pain, 48
   nausea and vomiting, 47
   swollen feet, 47–8
   toxaemia, 52
   varicose veins, 49
Procaine penicillin, use and dosage, 98
Prostate gland, enlarged, 45
Pulse, finding, 13–14
Pulse rate, 3, 4, 9
Pupils of eyes
   difference in size, 81
   reaction to light, 4

Rabies, 38–9
Radius, fractures, 77
Rehydration fluid, 41, 66
   use and dosage, 98
Respiration, 4
   rate, 3, 9
   see also Breathing
Respiratory arrest, 9
Ribs, fractures, 21, 77–8
Road accidents, prevention, 96

Scalds, see Burns and scalds
Scorpion stings, 36–7
   allergic reaction to antivenom, 24
Sedative poisoning, 33
Shell-fish, food poisoning from, 37
Shock
   checks for, 2
   effect on pain perception, 5
   from burns, 27
   from lightning strikes, 69
   priority actions, 6
   signs and symptoms, 6
   treatment, 6–7
Shoulder blade, fracture, 78–9
Sick feeling, see Nausea; Vomiting
Skin, 3
   colour, 4, 9
   damage from lightning strikes, 69

Skull fracture, 72–3
  causing bleeding from ear and nose, 82, 83
Snake bites, 35–6
  allergic shock from antivenom, 24
Sodium chlorate poisoning, 34
Spider bites, 37
Spinal injuries, 74–5
Splinting, 71
  using local plants, 72
Sprains, 80
Sternum, *see* Breast bone
Stomach, 3
Stomach ache, 40–6
  degree of pain, 40
Strains, muscular, 80
Stretchers
  blanketing, 87–8
  carrying, 90–2
  crossing stream, 93
  crossing uneven ground, 92
  crossing wall, 93
  improvising, 92
  loading, 88–90
  preparation, 87
  unloading, 92
Stroke, 6
  loss of consciousness due to, 30–1
Strychnine poisoning, 33
Suffocation, 7
Sulphadiazine, use and dosage, 98
Swelling, 5
  during pregnancy, 51–2
  from snake bites, 35
Symptoms, definition, 3

Teaching aids, 99–101
Temperature
  raised, cause of fits, 5
  reading thermometers, 3
  *see also* Cold, problems of; Heat, problems of
Tetanus
  allergic shock from antitetanus vaccine, 24
  cause of respiratory arrest, 7
  causing fits, 62–4
  in the newborn, 62–3
  protection against, 23
  test, 64
Tetracycline, use and dosage, 98
Thermometers, 3
Tibia, fractures, 79
Tongue, bleeding from, 84
Tooth socket, bleeding from, 84
Toxaemia of pregnancy, 52
Transport
  arranging, 7
  follow-up care during, 8
  methods, 85–93
  of patients with fractures, 75–6
  principles, 85
Two-handed seat, 86–7

Ultra, fractures, 77
Urinary system, 3
  infection, 44

Vaccination, antitetanus, 23–4
  allergic shock from, 24
Varicose veins, during pregnancy, 49
Vascular system, 3
Veins, 3
  bleeding, 17
  varicose, 49
Vomiting, 5
  during pregnancy, 47
  to relieve poisoning, 32–3

Weedkiller poisoning, 34
Witchcraft, loss of consciousness due to, 29
Worms, 42
Wounds, 17–25
  abdominal, 20
  aims of first aid, 17
  care, 18–23
  causes of infection, 23
  chest, 20
  crushed chest, 21
  dirty, special care of, 23
  flail chest, 21–2
  infection
    after stitching, 20
    treatment, 24–5
  local cures, 23
  penetrating, 20
  signs of infection, 24
  *see also* Cuts; Injuries